KT-154-882

Tower Hamlets College
Learning Centre

121577

Withdrawn

Knowledge Set

Medication

Debby Railton

THE LIBRARY
TOWER HAMLETS COLLEGE
POPLAR HIGH STREET
LONDON E14 0AF
Tel: 0207 510 7763

www.harcourt.co.uk

✓ Free online support
✓ Useful weblinks
✓ 24 hour online ordering

01865 888118

Heinemann

From Harcourt

Class: 615 · LMT
Accession No: 121
Type: Book

Heinemann, Halley Court, Jordan Hill, Oxford OX2 8EJ

Heinemann is the registered trademark of Harcourt Education Ltd

© Harcourt Education Ltd

First published 2007

12 11 10 09 08 07
10 9 8 7 6 5 4 3 2 1

British Library Cataloguing in Publication Data is available
from the British Library on request.

10-digit ISBN: 0 435 40231 5
13-digit ISBN: 978 0 43540231 0

Copyright notice
All rights reserved. No part of this publication may be reproduced
in any form or by any means (including photocopying or storing it
in any medium by electronic means and whether or not transiently
or incidentally to some other use of this publication) without the
written permission of the copyright owner, except in accordance
with the provisions of the Copyright, Designs and Patents Act
1988 or under the terms of a licence issued by the Copyright
Licensing Agency, 90 Tottenham Court Road, London W1T 4LP.
Applications for the copyright owner's written permission should
be addressed to the publisher.

Typeset by TexTech International Private Ltd
Printed by Ashford Colour Press Ltd
Illustrated by Sam Thompson/Calow&Craddock and TexTech
International Private Ltd
Cover design by David Poole
Cover photo: © Lottie Davies/Flowerphotos

Websites
Please note that the examples of websites suggested in this book
were up to date at the time of writing. We have made all links
available on the Heinemann website at www.heinemann.co.uk/
hotlinks. When you access the site, the express code is 2315P.

Contents

Introduction   iv

1. Legislation and medication   2

2. Roles, responsibilities and boundaries   14

3. Types of medicine and routes of administration   40

4. Safe practice in the administration of medicines   54

Trainer notes and guidance   74

Student log   92

Appendix 1
Blank MAR chart   98

Appendix 2
Blank prescription   99

Appendix 3
Staff drug audit template   100

Glossary   103

Index   105

Introduction

Knowledge sets have been created by Skills for Care and Development, part of the sector skills council. The idea behind each knowledge set is to provide key learning outcomes for specific areas of work within adult social care. This means that employers and training providers can use a knowledge set to provide in-house training as part of employees' continuing professional development. The advantage of using a knowledge set for the basis of training is that both employers and those who have undertaken training can be assured that a minimum standard has been reached. The knowledge sets also ensure consistency in knowledge and understanding across organisations and services.

The knowledge set for medication is aimed at those working in social care and handling medication. This book has been written by Debby Railton, an experienced pharmacist inspector with the Commission for Social Care Inspection. Using this book, in conjunction with the Skills for Care knowledge set, will:

- provide essential learning for all aspects of medicine management
- improve practice in order to meet the individual needs of those who receive care
- support those completing NVQ and other training
- develop the skills and knowledge base of those involved in handling medication
- support transition between different service settings in the social care sector
- ensure up to date and good practice.

The book is divided into the four main areas of the knowledge set:

- Legislation and medication
- Roles, responsibilities and boundaries
- Types of medicine and routes of administration
- Safe practice in the administration of medicines

These sections are further broken down into manageable topics, with spreads covering one or more learning outcomes. The following features have been designed to enhance the learning experience:

Activities – completion of the suggested activities and tasks will develop understanding and skills.

Care scenarios – real-life situations allowing knowledge to be put into practice.

Look it up – pointers to recognised reference sources that allow comparison of current knowledge with accepted good practice. You may also be asked to investigate your care setting's current procedures and practices.

Reflection – explore your level of knowledge as well as your thoughts, actions and behaviours.

Remember – key concepts and facts are highlighted and reinforced.

Question check – test your understanding and recall of a topic.

Space has often been provided for note-taking or the completion of activities and tables, although a notebook or workbook can be used alongside this book in order to expand on certain areas.

This book not only covers the learning outcomes for those undertaking training, but also includes a section for those developing or leading training sessions. The Trainer notes provide the answers to Care scenarios, guidance on the completion of activities and also expands on the knowledge given in the four main knowledge set areas. In addition, guidance on activities within the book often include ideas and suggestions for developing an activity and expanding on learning opportunities. Useful icons appear with each activity guidance feature, suggesting how long to spend on the activity and any materials that will be needed (e.g. flip chart, OHP, reference sources).

The Student log section of this book details all four main areas of the knowledge set for medication, along with the learning outcomes. Space is provided for trainees to log their progress and record those learning outcomes they have covered. In addition, the tables can also be used to map the content of this book against NVQ courses and any other relevant training being undertaken.

Used either as part of a training package or own its own by an individual, this *Knowledge set for medication* will prove to be an invaluable resource for those developing their career in the adult social care sector.

Acknowledgements

Harcourt would like to thank Skills for Care for giving permission to reproduce the tables of learning outcomes used in the student log section of this book (see pages 92–97).

The publisher and author would like to thank Jenny Chen, Education and Development Manager at The Bath Royal United Hospital, for her constructive review of this book.

The author would like to thank Morag Ross for her contributions to this book.

Photos

Gary Roebuck/Alamy, p46; Harcourt Education Ltd/Gareth Boden, p63; Mediscan, p4; Paul Doyle/Photofusion, p8; Richard Smith, p32.

1

Legislation and medication

1.1 Be aware of the legislation and guidance that controls the prescribing, dispensing, administration, storage and disposal of medicines

What you need to learn:

- legislation relating to medicines
- acts relating to your practice at work
- the Care Standards Act 2000
- patient records and confidentiality
- the administration and control of medicines in care homes.

Legislation relating to medicines

This section will lead you through the relevant legislation and guidance that controls prescribing (the doctor writing a prescription), dispensing (the pharmacist making up and giving out the medicines according to the prescription), administration (the care worker giving the medicines to individuals), storage (keeping the medicines safe) and disposal of medicines (getting rid of them once they are no longer needed).

Acts and Regulations relating to medicines are there to protect you and the individuals you look after. Some of the medicines might cause harm if handled inappropriately. Examples include spillages of medicines, injuries caused by needles and syringes, accidentally touching medicines used to treat cancer, applying creams and ointments and disposal of medicines the individual no longer needs. You should be provided with equipment to prevent or reduce any known risk of harm to you, your colleagues or the people you look after. This equipment may include gloves, aprons, washing facilities, spillage kits and sharps disposal containers.

Cleaning fluids may cause harm if misused by individuals in your care or if accidentally spilled. Information should be provided to tell you what to do if an accident occurs. Written documents relating to medicines given to individuals should be stored in a safe place and information shared with people that are responsible for the care of these individuals only.

Activity 1

Fill in the table below.

Why do you think acts and regulations exist?	
Who are they meant to protect?	
Name any acts or regulations that you may have heard of that relate in any way to medicines, cleaning fluids, records for medicine management, care plans.	

Legislation relating to medicines

Any person involved with medicines has to adhere to certain rules and regulations, whether this is the doctor, pharmacist or a person who administers them to other people. The following legislation controls prescribing, dispensing and storage of medicines.

The Medicines Act (1968)	This requires that the local pharmacist or dispensing doctor is responsible for supplying medication. He or she can only do this on the receipt of a prescription from an authorised person, for example, a doctor.
The Misuse of Drugs Act (1971)	This controls medicines that may cause harm if taken. These are called Controlled Drugs. The main purpose of this act is to prevent the misuse of these Controlled Drugs.
The Misuse of Drugs (Safe Custody) Regulations (1973)	This specifies how Controlled Drugs are to be stored and is referred to in the Standards for care homes. Controlled Drugs must be kept in a Controlled Drug cabinet that complies with these Regulations.

Legislation controlling the prescribing, dispensing and storage of medicines

Acts relating to your practice at work

These are written to protect the workforce from anything that may cause harm. Three are listed below that relate to medicines and cleaning fluids that you may use.

The Health and Safety at Work Act (1974)	This underpins regulations intended to reduce the risk posed by hazardous substances.
The Control of Substances Hazardous to Health Regulations (1999) (COSHH)	This requires employers to take all reasonable measures to protect their employees from any potentially dangerous substances or materials that they come into contact with whilst at work.
Hazardous Waste Regulations (2005)	This defines household and industrial waste and includes medicines that are no longer required. For example, care homes with nursing in England and Wales must use a clinical waste company to dispose of unwanted medicines. Other care homes can return medicines to the supplying pharmacy for destruction.

Acts relating to your practice at work

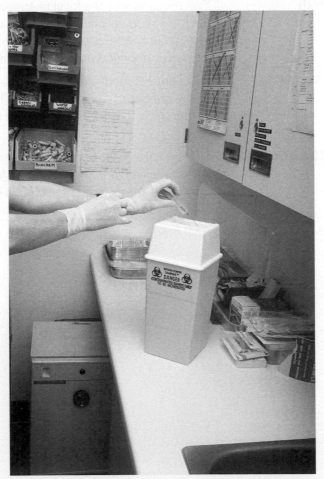

The Hazardous Waste Regulations (2005) control the disposal of clinical waste in your care setting

Activity 2

Think about substances that may cause harm. These include medicines and substances included under the COSHH regulations (for example, cleaning fluids). Fill in the table below.

Substance that may cause harm	Is it stored safely? Where?	What are the potential hazards if it is not stored safely and where would you get advice from if it is misused or spilt?

Care scenario: The 'strawberry milkshake'

The cleaner in a care home for people diagnosed with dementia had been provided with a big container of pink floor cleaner. This was far too big to pick up and use on a daily basis, so she decided to pour some of it into an empty bottle. She found an old empty four-pint plastic milk container and filled it with the cleaning fluid. One day, after a particularly busy morning, she left the milk container holding the pink floor cleaner on the table in the dining room. An individual came in and thought that it was some more of the strawberry milkshake that had been served the day before and drank the mixture. The individual became very ill and was rushed to hospital. Luckily, she had not drunk very much before a care assistant found her.

1. Under which act can the care home be prosecuted?
2. How could this situation have been avoided?

Activity 3

Fill in the table below.

Question	Answer/Comments
Do you have the product information available for all cleaning fluids?	
Where is the information kept? Alongside the substance that may cause harm (for example, the cleaning fluid) or in the office?	
Is it easy to find and read in an emergency?	

The Care Standards Act 2000

This legislation controls and promotes good practice in care services registered under the act. If your care service is registered under the Care Standards Act 2000, you will be expected to reach National Minimum Standards (NMS) to meet the needs of the individuals in your care.

The NMS are service specific, for example, Older People, Younger Adults, Domiciliary care. The Care Home Regulations 2001 and the Care Standards Act 2000 underpin these. It is important that you know the NMS relevant to the service you provide, to help you to meet the needs of the individuals who you look after.

You should be provided with a copy of the NMS relevant to your care service. The Commission for Social Care Inspection (CSCI) is the regulatory body which inspects care services for compliance with the National Minimum Standards and their accompanying regulations. The CSCI inspectors focus on the achievable outcomes for individuals. They will measure your service's performance against the Standards. Regulation 13(2) underpins the Standards about medicines and their uses and is mandatory, meaning that failure to meet this Regulation could result in prosecution.

The Mental Capacity Act 2005

This details that:

- an individual is assumed to have capacity to make a decision regarding their care
- a lack of capacity must be clearly demonstrated
- you must take all reasonable steps to help the individual make a decision. For example, using counselling or changing the formulation to help an individual take their medication
- an unwise decision by an individual does not mean they lack capacity to make a decision
- if it has been decided that an individual lacks the capacity to make a decision about their medication, any further decision made on their behalf must be made in their best interest (i.e. not the interests of the care staff, for example)
- the individual's rights and freedom of action must be taken into account. The decision taken should show that the least restrictive option or intervention is achieved. For example, it would not be acceptable to sedate an individual in order to stop them wandering around the care home.

Activity 4

Look at the NMS for your service relating to medicines, for example, Standard 9 for Older People, Standard 20 for Younger Adults etc. Imagine you are an inspector who has come to assess the medicine management in your care service. Fill in the following table with the outcome and the Standard number, e.g. 9.1, 9.2, and think whether the service you provide meets these Standards.

The final column is for you to complete at the end of this book to see if your opinion has changed.

	(Complete this section now.) Do you think you have met the outcome and Standards?	(This section should be completed at the end of the training book.) Do you think now that you have met the outcome and Standards?
Outcome e.g. Standard 9 for Older People		
Standard		
e.g. 9.1		
e.g. 9.2		
e.g. 9.3		

Activity 5

Read the latest report of your care service for the standard for medication, and fill in the following table.

Question	Comments
(Answer this question now.) Do you think the report reflects practice within your care service?	
(Answer this question at the end of your training course.) Do you still think your inspection report reflects practice in your care service?	

Patient records and confidentiality

This legislation controls record keeping of clinical information for the individuals whom you look after.

There are two acts relating to patient records that are important to you as a care worker.

The Access to Health Records Act (1990)	This act defines who may see medical records. The individual may see his or her own medical records, but nobody else may see them without permission from that individual. This includes next of kin and friends.
The Data Protection Act (1998)	This act applies to any organisation that keeps personal records on computer. They must: • be secure • allow the individual to have access to their records • record only relevant information • be used and disclosed only for its stated purpose.

Acts relating to patient records

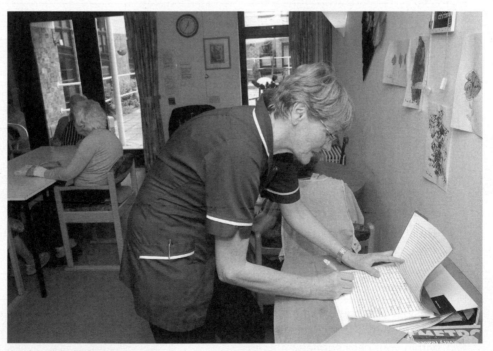

Keeping clinical information confidential is a very important part of your job

Activity 6

Fill in the table below.

Question	Comments
How do you think these acts might affect you?	
Are all the medical records held in a secure place?	
Does everyone have access to computer records or only specific people who actually need to see them?	
Are the records password protected?	

What do you think is the importance of storing all medical notes and any other sensitive information correctly?

Write down which laws may be broken if you do not store them correctly or if you discuss them with people who are not privy to the information.

Care scenario: The handyman

The Medicine Administration Records Charts and Care Assessments for a respite care unit were always recorded on the computer. A new individual had come into the home for two weeks of respite care. The computer was not password protected and anyone could gain access to it. The handyman knew the individual and had always thought he was a little strange, so he decided to find out the individual's medical background. He was able to access all of the individual's medical history and found out that he suffered from an underlying mental condition. That night, the handyman told his friends at the local pub about the individual.

1. Has the care home broken the law? If so, in what way has it broken the law?
2. What law did the handyman break, and how?

Patient confidentiality will be discussed in more detail in section 2.5.

Would you like your personal details or those of a close relative to be read and discussed by anyone else who was not involved in your or their care?

The Administration and Control of Medicines in Care Homes and Children's Services guidance document

This was published by the Royal Pharmaceutical Society of Great Britain in June 2003. This should be at your place of work and your trainer should give you a copy, alternatively it can be downloaded from their website, which you can access by going to www.heinemann.co.uk/hotlinks and entering the express code 2315P. It contains information on prescribing, dispensing, administration, storage and disposal of medicines.

Activity 7

Read a copy of the document detailed above and write down your thoughts about your practice. You should review these answers at the end of this book and write your thoughts at that time in the final column.

You should also look at this throughout the book and reflect on the good practice in each section for each learning outcome.

Think about the following questions and record your comments and thoughts about the guidance documents and your practice.

1. Do you follow the good practice?
2. Could improvements be made?

Section in the administration and control of medicines in care services and children's services	Thoughts before the course	Thoughts after the course
Policies and procedures		
Record keeping		
Medicines supply		
Storage of medicines		
Administration of medicines		
Disposal of medicines		
Controlled drugs		

Activity 8

Think of any activities you may have carried out recently which involved any of the acts, regulations and guidance documents you have looked at so far in this book. Are there any ways in which you might be able to improve your practice?

1. Why do you think there are acts, regulations and guidance documents?

2. Write down the acts, regulations and guidance documents relating to medicines.

3. Identify ways in which you think you can improve your practice.

1.2 Understand the legal framework and how the organisation's policies and procedures reflect these, for safe handling of medicines (prescribing, dispensing, administration, storage and disposal) by all care workers

This section will outline the legal framework for the safe handling of medicines and how the organisation's policies and procedures reflect these. This includes prescribing, dispensing, administration, storage and disposal of medicines by all staff responsible for medication management within their care practice.

Policies and procedures

The National Minimum Standards require that the registered person makes sure there is a policy for the receipt, recording, storage, handling, administration and disposal of medicines. They should promote the safety and well-being of the individuals whom you care for and also the safe practices of all care home staff.

A good policy should be written just for your place of work. You should be able to undertake any duties relating to medicines by reading the policy. It should guide you through exactly what to do from ordering the medicines to storage, administration and finally disposal of unwanted medicines.

Care scenario: The medicine mix-up

A care assistant did not follow her care home's procedure for administering medicines safely to one individual in her care. She gave someone else's medicine to this individual. There was no clear guidance in the medication policy as to what to do if this happened. The care assistant did not report the incident to anyone until the manager came on duty the next morning. By that time the drug administration error had caused serious harm to the individual.

1. How could this situation have been prevented?

Think about the care scenario (left). Does your medication policy give you guidance on what to do if this should happen to you, namely giving someone else's medicine to the wrong individual? Does your policy guide you through the correct procedures to follow to handle medication safely?

Do you understand the need for policies and procedures?

Who are they designed to protect?

Activity 9

Read the medication policies and procedures in your place of work.

Complete the following questions. As before, your answers should be reviewed at the end of this book.

Do they tell you how to	Yes/no (fill in now)	Yes/no (fill in at end of course)
Order medicines?		
Record the receipt of medicines?		
Record verbal orders? (Directions spoken to you personally by another health care professional over the telephone which have not been written down on a prescription.)		
Administer medicines?		
Store the medicines and ensure that the keys to the medication room, cabinet and medicine trolleys are kept in a safe place?		
Carry out processes concerning Controlled Drugs?		
Dispose of the medicines?		
Follow procedures if things go wrong?		
Administer home remedies? (Medicines that you can give out against a specific protocol, that the doctor has not prescribed.)		
Assess individuals for self administration?		
Handle medicines following the death of an individual?		
Handle oxygen supplies, emergency medicines and medicines an individual may need to take if he or she goes out on a trip away from home, and any specialist administration techniques?		
Record individuals' consent to medicines?		

1. Do you feel they include the current legislation around the safe handling of medicines to protect you and the individual from any harm?
2. Are they written just for your place of work? Do they name the doctors, pharmacies and contact information for other health care professionals?
3. Overall, do you think they are good, user-friendly policies/procedures?

Roles, responsibilities and boundaries

2.1 Understand the process by which medicines are prescribed, dispensed and obtained by the individual and the worker's role in the process

By the end of this section you should be able to understand the process by which medicines are prescribed, dispensed and obtained for the individual. You will also learn about your role and the roles of other healthcare professionals in this process.

People employed in social care have definite roles and responsibilities. It is important that you understand these roles and boundaries and what their responsibilities are. Specific titles may be given to certain jobs in the care service that you work in, but the table in the activity on page 15 lists the people commonly involved in care. Some will have direct involvement in the clinical care of the individuals, for example, administering the medicines to the individual; others will have indirect roles, for example, collecting the prescriptions from the surgery. All are important to ensure each individual's needs are met.

Care scenario: Staff shortages

A domiciliary care agency contracted to provide care to individuals who still live in their own homes was experiencing severe staff shortages. The clerical assistant at the agency was sent out to provide personal care to an individual. This was not within her job description and she had not been trained to undertake these roles. One task was to administer the medicines to the individual.

Unfortunately, she forgot to do this and the individual did not receive her routine pain relieving tablets. Because of this, the individual did not sleep well that night as she was in pain. A complaint was made to the Commission for Social Care Inspection (CSCI) and it was upheld. Evidence was found of staffing shortages and a lack of staff training. This was not the first time this situation had been identified. The domiciliary care agency received a Statutory Requirement Notice detailing the poor practice and what they had to do to improve the service to reach the required standards and meet the regulations. They failed to do this and the agency was prosecuted.

1. Why did the domiciliary care agency receive a Statutory Requirement Notice?
2. What should the agency have done to prevent this situation happening?

Activity 10

Complete the table below and fill in the names of people responsible in your own care service. Remember that titles may vary, but the general job description is probably the same.

Title	Definition	Names of the relevant people in your care service
Prescriber	The person who can legally diagnose and prescribe medicines. Examples include the general practitioner (GP) or doctor, dentist, some nurses and some pharmacists.	
Pharmacist	The person who dispenses and supplies the medicines and possibly Medication Administration Record (MAR) charts.	
District or community nurse	The person responsible for providing nursing assistance to people living in the community. (He or she may be able to prescribe some medicines.)	
Registered manager	The person who takes full responsibility for any action that occurs in the care service that is registered under the Care Standards Act. This includes all the processes that happen regarding medication. He or she may delegate this responsibility but remains ultimately responsible.	
Social care staff	These are usually the people that can administer the medicines in care services without nursing. They may each take responsibility for some or all of the following tasks: ordering, receipt, storage and disposal of medicines.	
Designated member of staff	There may be a specific person or people who are responsible for the whole process of medicine management in the care service.	
Ancillary staff	These are usually untrained staff who have no responsibility for medicine management. Some may undertake personal care, which may involve application of creams, for example. Specific tasks must be undertaken by them only if they have been trained to do so.	
Clerical staff/ administrators	These may deal with filing of MAR charts, arranging doctors' appointments and training sessions, and other routine clerical work. They would not be expected to handle any medication.	

2.2 Understand the roles and boundaries of all workers with regard to the safe handling of medicines (prescribing, dispensing, administration, storage and disposal) in various care contexts

By the end of this section you will understand the roles and boundaries of all workers with regard to the safe handling of medicines within various areas. These include, for example, care homes (with or without nursing), day services, individuals' own homes, sheltered accommodation, supported living, and other networks and services.

The table below lists the people who may handle medicines in different care contexts.

Type of service	Who can handle medicines
Care homes with nursing	Only registered nurses can handle and administer medicines in care homes with nursing.
Care homes without nursing	All staff must have successfully completed accredited training. These staff should be able to demonstrate the basic knowledge of how medicines are used, what they do and be able to recognise and deal with problems they may see relating to medication and understand and follow the principles behind all aspects of their home's policies on medicines-handling and records.
Domiciliary care	Individuals looked after in their own homes, receiving domiciliary care, which may involve care assistants taking responsibility for the individuals' medicine management. All staff must have received any necessary specialist training.
Residential special schools	Appropriate designated staff who must have received any necessary specialist training. Written authorisation by a doctor or nurse is required if medical or nursing procedures are carried out by school staff.
Children's homes	Competent designated staff monitored by a designated senior member of staff. All staff must have received any necessary specialist training. Written authorisation by a doctor or nurse is required if medical or nursing procedures are carried out by school staff.
Day services	There is no guidance (for example, National Minimum Standards), but it is advised that there should be a designated member of staff responsible for medication.
Sheltered accommodation	There is no guidance (for example, National Minimum Standards), but it is advised that there should be a designated member of staff responsible for medication.

People who handle medicines in different care contexts

Activity 11

Question	Comments
Are you aware of staff competencies and their specific roles?	
Are you confident that you only undertake tasks that you are trained to do and that are within your own competencies?	

Activity 12

Question	Comments
Do you understand the roles and boundaries of all workers with regard to the safe handling of medicines in the various care services? Think who works with you. Make a list of their role and their responsibilities. Check with them afterwards.	
Do you understand the legislation supporting the care services? (Look at section 1.1 starting on page 2 again) Write down how they apply to you.	
Do you feel confident that the people who handle medicines in your care service do so within their competence and have been trained to do so? If you don't, why not? What further training could be sought, and by whom?	

Think about the care service you work in and who looks after the individuals' medication. Look at the table on page 16 and see which service you provide (if it is listed there). Do you think medicine management varies between services? Or do you think basic principles apply?

2.3 Understand the need to check that the medicine received matches the medication and dosage prescribed by the clinician and is listed on the appropriate documentation

By the end of this section you should understand the need to check that the medicine received matches the medication and dosage prescribed by the clinician (for example, doctor, dentist) and is recorded on appropriate documentation.

This section will be broken down into six different areas:

- the prescription
- ordering prescriptions
- receipt of medicines
- the Medicine Administration Record (MAR) chart
- new individuals' medications
- verbal orders.

Activity 13

Look at a prescription written for you or an individual and complete the table below.

Does it have the following?	Yes	No
Name and address of the patient		
Age and/or date of birth		
The name of the medicine and its formulation (for example, tablets, mixture)		
The strength and dose		
The quantity		
The date		
The name and address of the prescribing doctor, dentist, or nurse or pharmacist		
The signature of the prescriber (it must be signed to make it valid)		

The prescription

The majority of medicines administered by carers will be prescribed by a clinician, for example, a doctor, dentist or in some instances a nurse or pharmacist, and then dispensed by a community or hospital pharmacist, or dispensing doctor. You must administer the medicines exactly as they are written on the prescription at all times.

Prescription jargon

Doctors used to write prescriptions in Latin, and many directions today are still written in Latin, although they use abbreviated versions. Listed below are some common abbreviations you may see on a prescription. Fill in the following table, writing in the directions in English (the back of the British National Formulary (BNF) has a list that may help you).

A prescription for any medicine written by a clinician is valid for 13 weeks from the date it was written unless it is a prescription for Controlled Drugs, where it is valid for 28 days from the date it was written.

Latin Abbreviation	Direction
o.d.	
b.d.	
t.d.s., t.i.d.	
q.d.s., q.i.d.	
qqh	
a.c.	
p.c.	
cc	
p.r.n.	
mane or o.m.	
nocte or o.n.	
m.d.u.	
stat	
I.U	
mg	
mcg	
ml	
p.o.	
i/m	
i/v	
neb.	
Guttae or G	
Oint or Oc	
elix.	

Common prescription abbreviations

If you are responsible for the individuals' medicines within the service you provide, you are responsible for signing the back of the prescription and ticking the reason for exemption from prescription charges. Proof of exemption may be required at the pharmacy.

Medicines prescribed for an individual are their property. The Medicines Act (1968) states that each medicine must only be administered to the person for whom they have been prescribed, labelled and supplied. This means that prescribed medication cannot be used as 'stock' and administered to any individual other than whom they are prescribed to. This includes dressings, nutritional supplements, catheters, etc.

The Medicines Act (1968) also allows the administration of a prescribed medicine by you, a third party (not the clinician or the individual), in accordance with the prescription for that person (except injections). This enables you to administer medicines to individuals in your care.

Care scenario: Joe

Joe is looked after at home and the domiciliary care staff are responsible for collecting his prescription from the doctor and getting the medicines dispensed at the pharmacy. A care assistant picked up the prescription and took it in to her local pharmacy the next day, ready to take along to the next appointment with Joe. However, the pharmacist was unable to dispense the prescription because the doctor had not signed it. The care assistant therefore had to take it back to the surgery to be signed, delaying her subsequent appointments.

1. How could the care assistant have avoided this situation?
2. What could the care service have done to avoid this happening?

Activity 14

Question	Comments
Write a list of all the details that must be written on the prescription.	
Whose responsibility is it to sign for an exemption of the prescription tax if you are in charge of an individual's medicine?	
Do you work for a domiciliary care service? If so, does the pharmacist collect from the surgery, dispense the prescription and deliver the medicines to individuals, or do you do this? Why should the pharmacist not give this service for a care home?	

Ordering prescriptions

Activity 15

Fill in the final column of the following table with notes about your practice.

Task	Notes	Your practice and comments
Identify the medicines that need to be ordered	The majority of medicines are repeat prescriptions.	
Request the prescription from the surgery	Ask for sufficient quantities to last the 28-day cycle (7 days in some instances).	
Check the prescription received against the old MAR chart	It is normally the duty of the receptionist in the surgery to generate these prescriptions. Their correct production depends upon the information stored in the doctor's computer. Errors may occur if changes that have been made to the individual's medication have not been updated on the computer, resulting in the old medication or dose being prescribed.	
Rectify any problems with the surgery before the prescription is dispensed	It is easier to correct any discrepancies with a prescription before it is dispensed.	
Photocopy the prescription to check the dispensed medicines and MAR chart against the prescription	A different procedure may be detailed in the medication policy. It must be robust enough to check the dispensed medicines and MAR chart with the original prescription for any discrepancies.	
Sign the back of the prescription and claim exemption if applicable Send the prescription to the pharmacy to be dispensed	Proof of exemption may be required.	
Check the dispensed medicines received and the MAR charts against the photocopied prescription Address any discrepancies or errors with the pharmacist before any administration takes place	Keep a photocopy of the prescription with the MAR chart for reference.	

(Continued)

Task	Notes	Your practice and comments
Record the quantity of medicines received on the MAR chart	The pharmacist may print the quantity he or she dispenses, but you should record the actual quantity you receive and/or balances carried over from previous months.	
Ensure a second member of staff confirms the accuracy of the MAR chart and medicines received	Both care assistants involved in the checking procedure should sign the MAR chart.	
Safely store all the medicines in a locked trolley or cabinet	Make sure the keys are kept in the sole possession of the person in charge and responsible for the administration of medication at the care home.	
Administer the medicines and record what happened	This will be discussed in more detail later (Medicine Administration Record charts, page 26).	

After a set period of time the whole process will start again. This is usually about week 3 of the cycle.

Care scenario: Once or twice a day?

A care home has received a delivery of medicines, but the senior carer did not check them in and instead just put them in the trolley for the next 28-day cycle. The doctor had changed the dose of one medicine from two tablets daily to one tablet daily. The MAR chart read two daily and the label on the bottle read one daily. It is now the weekend and the doctor's surgery is closed until Monday. The correct dose can therefore not be confirmed.

1. What should the home have done to prevent this situation happening?
2. How could this situation be avoided in the future?
3. Why is it important to avoid situations like this?

Think about the practice in your care service. Do you follow all the points in the table to obtain a supply?

Care scenario: Running out of medication

A doctor has written a prescription for the following medicines:

- aspirin 75mg x 28; one to be taken each morning
- furosemide 20mg x 28; one to be taken each morning
- nifedipine 20mg retard x 28; one to be taken twice a day.

The care service ran out of nifedipine and the individual went without the medication until a new supply was available. The doctor has written a 28-day supply for aspirin and furosemide but only a 14-day supply for nifedipine retard.

1. How could the staff have avoided this situation happening?
2. How could this be avoided in the future?

Does your medication policy reflect this good practice for checking the prescriptions and checking the dispensed medicines received into the home?

Does your care service follow best practice to ensure that all the medicines are received on time and at the correct dose and quantity?

What can you do to influence improvements which may save staff time and the quality of life for the service user to prevent medicines running out and having to be ordered mid-cycle?

Activity 16

Some common problems with ordering prescriptions are recorded below. Think of the possible reasons why these may happen and possible solutions. List any further problems that you have experienced personally.

Problems	Reasons	Solutions
Not obtaining prescriptions in time for the monthly order		
Running out of medicines mid-cycle		
Doses not specified and you don't know how to give them		
Pharmacist unable to supply a medicine		
You do not copy the prescription so cannot check the new medicines and MAR charts into the home properly		
The old dose is printed on the MAR chart and label even though the doctor changed the dose when he visited the home		

Receipt of medicines

Medicines must only be administered from pharmacist-labelled containers. All the dispensed medicines should be labelled. The pharmacist has to comply with the Medicines (Labelling) Regulations 1976, as amended. An example is shown below.

```
              15g Fucidin 2% cream
              Apply TWICE a day
              FOR EXTERNAL USE ONLY

Miss Joanne Brown                    09/06/06
Keep out of the reach of children
              BRIDGES Pharmacy
       Farmhouse Way, Littletown. Tel: 123456.
```

An example of a pharmacy label

The medicines will be dispensed into either traditional bottles or boxes or in Monitored Dosage Systems (MDS). These should be labelled as the clinician directs on the prescription. MDS can be used for certain formulations of medicines, for example, some tablets and capsules. These are dispensed in blister packs to aid administration by the individual or care staff. Various systems are available on the market, e.g. Manrex®, Venalink®, Nomad®.

The system supplied depends on what the pharmacist can offer, but the ultimate choice of what system suits the home is up to the staff or the individual receiving domiciliary care. It may be a 7-day or 28-day MDS for individual medicines or all the medicines dispensed together in a blister for each time of day.

MDS can only be used for solid oral dose medicines. Liquids, inhalers, eye drops, creams, effervescent tablets and certain tablets or capsules with known stability problems cannot be dispensed into MDS. This results in two different systems of medicine administration being used in the home (MDS and containers). This may cause problems if protocols for administration are not followed. These will be discussed later in section 4.4, pages 60–1.

The expiry date is shorter, usually 8 weeks, once medicines are dispensed in MDS. This may result in an increase in medicine waste (particularly for 'when required' (PRN) medication where the medicine is not given routinely at set times each day but only occasionally).

All MDS must be labelled in the same way as a traditional container each time they are dispensed. Tablets or capsules which cannot be identified and are similar to each other should not be placed together in a MDS. All medicines must be identifiable and the description labelled by the pharmacist.

Under the Disability and Discrimination Act 2005 (DDA) pharmacists may assess the individual and decide whether he or she qualifies to have his or her medicine dispensed in a compliance aid, for example, an MDS where the medicines are dispensed in a daily container or blister pack. If they are being looked after by care assistants, for example, in domiciliary care, they may not qualify to have their medicines dispensed in an MDS, as trained staff are responsible for administering the medicines and not the individuals themselves. Care homes may have an agreement with the pharmacist that they wish their medicines to be dispensed in MDS.

The pharmacist has to label the medicine following the directions recorded on the prescription. It is advisable in care services that the instruction 'as directed' is avoided. Full directions of how the doctor wishes the medicines to be used or administered should be specified on the prescription so the pharmacist can label it as the doctor intended.

What does the pharmacist dispense the medicines into for your service? Is this referred to in the medication policy?

Care scenario: Jane

Jane was recently prescribed an antibiotic for a chest infection. The doctor told the care assistant on duty that it should be given four times a day, and handed her a prescription recording the instructions 'as directed'. The care assistant was going on holiday for a few days and dropped the prescription off at the local pharmacy on her way home from work. The pharmacy labelled the medicine and delivered it to the home. It was not dispensed into the MDS used by the home. The following problems then occurred.

- The new care assistant on duty did not know what the doctor had told the previous care assistant, and decided to administer the antibiotic three times a day.
- As the doses were not in the MDS, many were not administered, as staff did not look at the MAR chart before they administered the medicines.
- Jane's chest infection did not get better and the doctor was called after 10 days.
- He prescribed a different antibiotic to treat the infection.

1. What procedure should the first care assistant have followed to avoid this situation? (This will be discussed in more detail on page 32 – verbal orders.)
2. When should the second care assistant have contacted the doctor to check the dose?
3. How should the MAR chart have helped to enable correct administration of the medicine?
4. What alterations or notes (if any) should have been made to the MAR chart?
5. How could the medicines dispensed in a different system (i.e. traditional containers instead of MDS) be identified on the MAR chart to remind staff that these also have to be administered?

Activity 17

Look at the medicines in your care service and answer the questions in the following table.

Question	Comments
Are all the medicines you administer labelled or have you thrown the labelled box away? What can be done to avoid this scenario?	
Can you identify all the medicines dispensed in the MDS?	
Look at two labels on two separate medicines for an individual. Do they record all the information needed to administer the medication safely or are the directions unclear, for example, 'as directed'? How could this situation be avoided?	

Care scenario: Peter

Peter has been prescribed Hydroxocobalamin injections. These are to be administered by the district nurse, who visits the care home every two months. The home is responsible for ordering the medication. Three ampoules were prescribed to be administered over the next six months. This was printed on the MAR chart the first month. However, it was not printed on subsequent MAR charts, as no prescription was ordered, so it was not dispensed. Staff also did not carry over the balance of the ampoules or flag up when the next dose was due to be administered.

1. Without the Hydroxocobalamin recorded on the next month's MAR chart, was this the complete record of all Peter's medicines?
2. What should the staff have recorded, and why?
3. What should they do if the nurse fails to visit for the next injection?

Care scenario: Eric

Eric has had his blood levels taken to calculate the dose of warfarin he needs. His warfarin dose changes after every blood test. Staff are finding it difficult to record the correct dose on the MAR chart. Three strengths of warfarin were recorded on the MAR chart and were available to administer in the trolley, despite the dose always being below 4 mg. Gaps were common and it could not be proven whether the dose had been given or even what dose had been administered.

1. What could be done to correct the situation?
2. What would be the effect on Eric's health of the administration of the incorrect dose of warfarin?

Activity 19

Eric's warfarin dose has just changed from 3 mg, 2 mg alternate days to 3 mg on weekdays and 2 mg at the weekend.

Complete a blank MAR chart, indicating when the warfarin must be administered. Record the old dose for one week from 01/03/06 until 08/03/06 and then the new dose from 09/03/06.

Note: staff have recorded the quantities (Q) received, together with the date.

1. Why is the MAR chart such an important document?
2. What specific information must a MAR chart record?
3. How should it be used to check the new prescriptions before they are dispensed?
4. How should you record the quantities of any medicines carried over to the next 28-day cycle on the new MAR chart?
5. How could you identify, on the MAR chart, medicines that are dispensed in a traditional container, if the majority of medicines are dispensed in MDS?
6. Where is the best place to keep a copy of the prescription so all staff who administer the medicines can see it?

Does your medication policy state that:

- all prescribed medication must be recorded on the MAR chart?
- medicines for occasional use and any carry-over balances must be recorded?
- the MAR chart should be used to check the prescriptions before they are dispensed?
- the new MAR chart and dispensed medicines should be checked against a copy of the prescription?

Care scenario: Freadah

A doctor had visited Freadah, who lived in a care home, just after the medicines had been ordered. He saw Freadah and changed her dose of hypnotic (sleeping tablet) from two tablets each night to one each night, because she was feeling very drowsy in the mornings and was unsteady on her feet. Unfortunately the doctor didn't change the information on the computer at the surgery.

The new prescriptions for the following 28-day cycle were written and signed by another doctor in the practice. The home didn't check the new prescriptions against the MAR chart before they were sent to the pharmacy, and did not notice that Freadah had been prescribed the old dose regime of two tablets at night.

The new MAR charts were printed and the tablets dispensed. No checks were made upon receipt and Freadah was administered the old dose of hypnotic. Four days later Freadah stood up to get a biscuit, felt dizzy and fell over. She broke her hip and was admitted to hospital.

1. How could this situation have been prevented?

New individuals' medications

For each new individual who receives care from you, you must take steps to check all his or her medicines you receive and that it is his or her current medicine regime.

This can be confirmed from:

- a discharge prescription from the hospital
- a repeat prescription copy brought in by the individual
- the pre-admission assessment by another health care professional.

If there is no means to confirm the individual's current medication, you must make contact with his or her doctor to confirm you have all the prescribed medication at the right doses, to administer. This must be done at the earliest opportunity and you must record you have done this. You should never assume that the medication brought in by the individual or his or her relatives is their current drug regime without written confirmation to support it.

Activity 20

Write down what steps you take to confirm the drug regime for new individuals who have come to live in your care service.

_____

_____

_____

_____

1. Have you provided evidence that you have confirmed the individual's current medication regime?
2. How should communication be documented and kept?
3. Do you have a template specifically for recording the individual's medication and with whom you confirm this?

Care scenario: Mohammed

Mohammed was due to go into a care home for two weeks of respite care. His son brought in his medicines, having collected them from the medicine cabinet at his father's home. He didn't know that his father suffered from epilepsy and that he kept his medication for that in a different place. Staff failed to check Mohammed's current medication regime with the doctor and administered only the medicines that his son had brought in.

After five days, Mohammed had an epileptic fit and the doctor was called. The doctor asked if Mohammed had taken his anti-epileptic medication. The care staff said that they did not know Mohammed was an epileptic or that he was meant to be taking prescribed medication to prevent epileptic fits.

1. What procedures should the staff have followed and when to prevent this situation?

Does your care home's medication policy include how to confirm individuals' medications received into the care service before you administer it?

1. Why is it important to verify the current drug regime?

2. Whom could you contact to get this information?

3. What written sources of information could you use to verify this?

4. What could happen to an individual if you did not do this?

5. Do you have a template to record verbal confirmation of a drug regime?

Activity 21

Create a template to record verbal confirmation of a medicine regime.

Verbal orders

Occasionally a doctor may change the dose of a medication halfway through a 28-day cycle. They may do this verbally, meaning that a second prescription may not be written. You should have a written protocol and template to prompt you to record all the information from the doctor accurately.

The verbal dose change should be recorded immediately. It should include the following:

- the date and time
- the doctor's name
- the individual's name
- the name of the medicine
- the new dose and frequency
- any special instructions
- the name of the person who recorded the information.

This information should be repeated back to the doctor to confirm you have recorded it correctly, and then written on the MAR chart signed and dated. It should be checked by a second member of staff for accuracy and signed. This should be recorded as a separate entry and the old dose crossed out and dated.

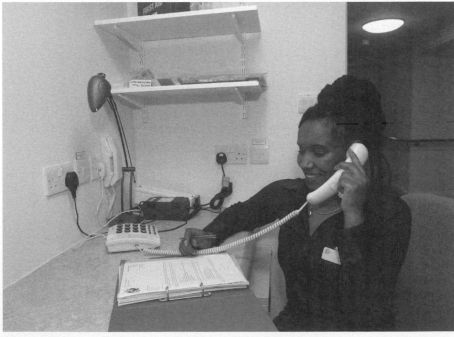

A doctor may change an individual's medication over the phone

What procedures do you follow when the clerk from the doctor's surgery phones through a dose change of a medicine prescribed at a clinic in a hospital? For example, what if he or she advises you of an INR result and changes a warfarin dose?

Always try to obtain written confirmation of any dose change following a verbal instruction as soon as possible, for example, a fax from the doctor detailing the dose change.

Care scenario: Jonathan

Jonathan has attended a warfarin clinic and the care home is waiting to hear from the clinic regarding the new dose. The secretary at the care home takes the call from the warfarin clinic and writes the new dose down on a scrap of paper. The secretary gives the piece of paper to a care assistant, who changes the dose as written on the paper. Unfortunately, the secretary is not trained to handle medication instructions and did not understand the complex dose change. The warfarin dosage was therefore written down incorrectly. As a result, Jonathan was administered the wrong dose.

A few days later, Jonathan fell over and cut himself. It was difficult to stop the bleeding, and it was decided to call for an ambulance to take him to hospital. Following an investigation, it became clear that the wrong dose of warfarin had been administered, because it had been incorrectly written on the MAR chart. This was a direct consequence of the care staff failing to follow procedures of good practice for verbal instructions.

1. Who should take verbal information regarding medication?
2. How should verbal instructions be recorded to ensure all the relevant information is included?
3. How can the accuracy of verbal instructions be checked?

Activity 22

Use the template created in Activity 21 on page 31 to record a verbal order from a colleague. Your trainer will help you to do this.

Do you have set procedures and a template to record them, within your care service, for receiving verbal orders and instructions? Can this be implemented in your service if you do not?

By the end of this section you should understand the need to seek guidance and support about the medicines and dosages prescribed for individuals in your care.

> Do not forget other sources of information. If you do use them, do not forget to document what advice they give you in the individuals' personal records. Possible other sources of information are listed in the following table.

Source	Information provided
The individual	The individual is an important source of information regarding the medicines he or she takes. He or she is the one taking the medicines and has unique and important information about what he or she needs to take and why.
The clinician	The actual prescriber will be able to help you if you are unsure of anything that you administer. The clinician must be informed of any side effects or drug administration errors so that he or she is aware of exactly what the individual has been administered and what has happened following administration.
The pharmacist	The community pharmacist who supplies the actual medicines is specifically trained to know what all medicines do. If you have any query regarding the medicines you administer, you can discuss this with the pharmacist, who should be happy to advise you.
The district or community nurse	The district or community nurse is often an expert in many areas of products, for example, dressings, any injections they administer or inhaler use for asthma.
NHS Direct	This is a good source of information regarding any problems you may have with medication. It is an extremely useful point of contact for any 'out of hours' query that cannot be dealt with by your community pharmacist. They will advise you of the appropriate action to take in the event of an emergency or drug administration error.
Your manager	The registered person who is responsible for running the service you provide should also be aware of how to access information and where to seek additional guidance.

Other sources of information about medicines

Activity 23

There are a variety of reference sources available, giving current and relevant information about the medicines your individuals take. The following table lists good common sources of information. Compare information in each reference source for ibuprofen or a medicine of your choice.

Reference source	Where it is found	Record the following using each reference source for ibuprofen or a medicine of your choice			
		The adult dose	Two side effects	One drug interaction	One warning or caution
The British National Formulary (BNF)	This includes information about medicines, including their indications, dose ranges, side effects and possible drug interactions. It is updated every six months and it is important to use the current reference source for up-to-date information. Available from bookshops and online. Visit www.heinemann.co.uk/hotlinks for a link. Enter the express code 2315P.				
The MIMS (Monthly Index of Medical Specialities)	This contains information about drugs that are available on prescription or sold over the counter (GSL and P medicines). This can be purchased from good bookshops.				
The Product Information Leaflet (PIL)	This must be supplied by the pharmacist for each medicine dispensed. This is written by the drug manufacturer and explains all about the medicines, for example, how to take them, side effects, cautions, dose, etc. You could build your own portfolio of them, containing all the medicines you administer in your care service.				

Activity 24

An individual in your care has been taking atenolol for hypertension, furosemide for oedema (swelling) of his ankles and aspirin for prevention of myocardial infarction for a few weeks. He has recently developed a chest infection and was prescribed amoxicillin 250 mg, three times a day for 7 days. After two doses of amoxicillin, he developed a red rash all over his body. Answer the following questions.

Question	Answer
Using a good reference source, look up the four medicines and record which medicine may cause a rash: ■ atenolol ■ furosemide ■ aspirin ■ amoxicillin.	
Which medicine do you think may have caused the rash? (Consider when the rash appeared.)	
What would you do about it? Who should you contact immediately about the rash?	
Who else could you have contacted to seek information about the red rash?	

Care scenario: Mrs Ghuman's crocodile

Mrs Ghuman was prescribed Tramadol 100 mg four times a day for severe pain. She has recently been crying and complaining that she has a crocodile at the end of her bed that is waiting to eat her and that it is also following her around the home. Care staff thought this might be due to her underlying dementia and decided to inform the old-age psychiatrist at Mrs Ghuman's next appointment. A pharmacist visited the home during his routine visits and the care staff told him about Mrs Ghuman's recent behaviour. Tramadol was prescribed at the maximum daily dose of 400 mg and Mrs Ghuman was given it regularly for a few weeks. Looking at the MAR charts and daily records, the pharmacist tracked back to the time she started seeing the crocodile in her bedroom and linked this to the administration of Tramadol.

1. Look up the medicine Tramadol in a good reference source. What side effects are listed?
2. What action should the care staff take now the pharmacist has suggested a link between the medication and Mrs Ghuman's crocodile?

Activity 25

Think about the individuals in your care. Look up the usual doses and side effects for all the medicines one individual in your care is currently taking. Choose someone who is taking no more than four medicines.

Medicine and dose	Possible side effects	Does the individual experience any of these?

1. Do you talk to the individual about his or her medication and how they feel? Do you discuss with the individual any reasons why he or she refuses to take his or her medicines?
2. Do you feel confident about reporting any side effects to the doctor?
3. Could you discuss any problems found with the pharmacist instead?

Think about all the individuals in your care, and fill in the following table.

Question	Comments
Do you know the general indications (what they are for), doses and common side effects for all the medicines you administer?	
Do you have access to good reference sources?	
Do you discuss the individuals' medications with them?	
Can you confidently discuss the medicines and the effects they have on the individual with other members of your team and your manager?	
Where could you obtain additional medical information about the medicines?	
What would you do if you suspected that an individual was experiencing a side effect to a medicine?	

There are two acts that relate to patient records which are important to you as a care worker. You can refresh your memory by turning back to page 8 in section 1.1.

Confidentiality

It is important that you maintain the individual's confidentiality at all times. You should never talk about the individual's clinical condition or the medicines they take with anyone except the health care professionals involved in his or her care, unless you have the individual's written permission, given by the individual, to discuss these things with named people, for example, the individual's next of kin.

You are responsible for maintaining the confidentiality of the individual in your care and you are accountable for your actions if you do discuss the individual's condition and treatment with anyone else without the individual's consent.

If the individual cannot make his or her own informed decision about the care and medicines he or she receives, an advocate or solicitor with power of attorney may take responsibility for deciding what is in the best interest of the individual.

Care scenario: The notice board

The aunt of a 15-year-old girl who lived in a children's home was talking to the care staff about her niece. A prescription for the niece was pinned up on the notice board awaiting dispensing. It was for the contraceptive pill. The aunt noticed the prescription and was furious and said that her niece should not be encouraged to be sexually active, and subsequently complained about the girl's care to the manager of the children's home.

1. What acts did the children's home break, and what could this have led to?
2. Who suffered as a consequence of this event, and how?

Activity 26

Vera's daughter has recently visited her and asks you about the medication her mother is currently taking, as she has noticed that her mother is very drowsy and difficult to wake. Write down what you would do. Fill in the reflection box at the end of this section to see if your opinion has changed.

What would you do?	Reflection

Vera herself wishes to know what medicines she is now taking, as she does not feel very well since starting her new tablets. Do you think it is acceptable to show her notes and MAR chart to her?

Yes/no	Why?

Where do you store all the records within your care home? Are they secure or do other people have access to them?

Do your medication policies include a section on patient confidentiality? With whom are you able to discuss an individual's medications and clinical condition without breaching the law?

Go back to Activity 26 about Vera's daughter and reflect on your answers. Do you still agree with what you first wrote down?

1. How could you prevent unauthorised staff having access to medical records held in the home?

2. Are you confident that you do not talk about confidential information with people who have no right to know?

3. Do you secure all confidential information in a safe place that is not accessible to other individuals, staff and members of the public?

4. Do you think you have breached the laws of patient confidentiality by mistake?

5. If you have, what could you do so you do not do it again?

Types of medicine and routes of administration

3.1 Understand the importance of some types of medication prescribed and administered to individuals

As discussed in section 2.4, you need to be familiar with all the medicines you administer and what they are for. Access to information about the medicines is important, and recognising side effects and common doses is essential for good care of individuals.

- You should know what all the medicines you administer are for.
- You should know or have a reference source to identify common side effects.
- You should understand why you administer all the medicines you do.

Look at three MAR charts and test yourself about whether you know what each medicine is prescribed for and what it does. Look at an individual's care plan. Does this include information on the clinical conditions the individual has, and can you identify the medicines he or she is prescribed to treat it?

Do you feel confident that you know what each medicine you administer is for? Are you aware of their common side effects?

How do you think you can improve on your knowledge? Do you have adequate reference sources to check out what each medicine does?

Care scenario: Kathleen

Kathleen has been prescribed the following medication: Senna tablets (two at night), Lactulose syrup (15 ml twice a day) and Movicol sachets (one daily when required). Care assistants have been administering all three medicines every day. After a week or so, Kathleen began having mild diarrhoea. When this got quite bad, the care assistants stopped giving all of the medicines. Once Kathleen's diarrhoea stopped, they then started giving all three medicines again. This happened regularly throughout the 28-day cycle.

1. Why did Kathleen keep having diarrhoea on a regular basis?

Activity 27

Complete the following table and fill in the name of a medicine that you may have administered with the dose and common side effects. The first one has been filled in as an example.

You will have to use good reference sources, for example, the BNF, MIMS or any Product Information leaflets (PILs) (see page 35). The BNF index lists medical conditions and the medicines used to treat them. Try to give examples of medicines that you have actually administered to individuals.

Medicine for the treatment of:	Example	Common adult dose	Common side effects
chest infection	amoxicillin	250 mg three times a day	sickness, rash
allergies			
heartburn			
anticoagulation (to stop blood clots)			
depression			
not sleeping (insomnia)			
anxiety			
high blood pressure			
asthma			
sickness			
pain			
epilepsy			
diabetes			
Parkinson's disease			
dementia			
cancer			
anaemia			
inflammation			
eye infection			
fungal infection			
ear infection			
eczema			

By the end of this section you should understand the classification of medicines, for example: Prescription Only Medicines (POM), Pharmacy only medicines (P), General Sales List medicines (GSL), Controlled Drugs (CD) and herbal, homeopathic and complementary remedies. Controlled Drug records will be discussed here briefly, and in more detail on page 64.

- A *drug* is any substance which, when taken into the body, may modify one of its functions.
- A *medicine* is a drug that is used in the treatment or prevention of a disease. There are two names of medicines:
  - The *generic* (non-proprietary) name. This is based on the medicine's main ingredient, for example, paracetamol.
  - The *trade* or *brand* name. This is the manufacturer's name, for example, Panadol®.

Medicines are classified according to the Medicines Act (1968). Fill in two examples of each classification of medicine in the table below.

Classification	Abbreviation	Definition	Examples
General Sales List medicines	GSL	These must be licensed and are sold in shops, supermarkets, etc. and do not require a pharmacist to be present unless they are purchased from a pharmacy.	
Pharmacy only medicines	P	These can only be sold in registered pharmacies under the supervision of a pharmacist.	
Prescription Only medicines	POM	These must be prescribed before a pharmacist or dispensing doctor can supply them.	
Controlled Drugs	CD	These must be prescribed by a doctor. They have to be stored in a more secure cabinet and a record made in a Controlled Drugs register.	

Complementary or alternative medicines

These can be purchased from your local pharmacy, supermarket or health shop. A few may be prescribed by medical practitioners.

Homeopathic medicines

Homeopathy works by treating the whole person. Homeopathic remedies are believed to work by a principle of 'like curing like'. This means that a substance, which in high doses can cause harm, can cure the same symptoms when given in tiny doses. It is believed that the small dose stimulates the body to heal itself.

Herbal remedies

These can be prescribed by a herbal medical practitioner and are also available from health food shops and pharmacies. They should be used with caution in the elderly, pregnant women and breastfeeding women. Some are known to interact with traditional medicines, and advice should always be taken from a medical practitioner (doctor or the pharmacist) before any herbal remedy is administered. A common example is St John's wort when taken with some medicines used to treat epilepsy.

Chinese medicines

These are used to restore the imbalances in the body that have caused the disease. They are usually prescribed by a traditional Chinese medical practitioner, but some can be purchased over the counter.

Look up your care home's procedures for the handling of Controlled Drugs. Does it state that two people have to be involved in any procedure involving Controlled Drugs?

Activity 28

Gather together five medicines that you administer to individuals, which have been dispensed in the manufacturer's box. Look at the generic name and brand name, and also the classification of the medicine. Then fill in the table below.

Generic name	Brand name	Classification	Can you buy them in a shop or pharmacy, or do they have to be prescribed?

Controlled Drugs

These are classified according to the Misuse of Drugs Act (1971). They have certain restrictions about prescribing, storage and record keeping. Examples include temazepam, morphine, phenobarbitone, fentanyl, methylphenidate and diamorphine.

It is advised that all Controlled Drugs (CDs) are stored in a CD cabinet that complies with the Misuse of Drugs (Safe Custody) Regulations (1973). This is a double skinned metal cabinet with a double lock and an internal hinge. It should be rag bolted to a solid wall (not a partition wall). All transactions must be recorded in a CD register in addition to the MAR chart.

The CD register must be bound and have serial page numbers (page 1, 2, 3, etc., to make sure no pages are removed). Each transaction (for example, the administration or the receipt of these medicines) must be recorded by two people – the person undertaking the transaction and the person witnessing it. This is in addition to the care assistant recording the administration or receipt on the MAR chart. (This will be discussed in more detail on page 64.)

Do you know the difference between GSL, P and POM medicines, and CDs? Do you know the difference between traditional and complementary medicines? Can you list a commonly-used CD in your care service?

Do you record all CD transactions in the CD register? Are they always witnessed?

Does the CD register balance tally with that on the MAR chart?

In this section, the following routes to administer medicines will be discussed:

- ingestion (by mouth)
- inhalation
- injection
- topically
- infusion
- instillation
- rectally
- vaginally
- transdermally
- PEG (Percutaneous Endoscopic Gastrostomy) tube.

Ingestion (by mouth)

Medicines can be taken by mouth (either swallowed or sublingually – put under the tongue). The majority of medicines are formulated to be taken by mouth (orally) in the form of a tablet, capsule or liquid. They come in a variety of shapes and sizes, colours and tastes.

- *Solid dose oral formulations* are either made as tablets or capsules. Tablets or capsules may be formulated to slowly release the medicine and so, if released all at once, they may cause an overdose. If you crush tablets you may inhale fine particles of it, which may have an adverse effect on your health.

- *Liquids, oral solutions, suspensions and syrups* are measured using a 2.5 ml or 5 ml spoon, oral syringe or a medicine tot and are useful for children's medicines and for individuals with swallowing difficulties.

Crushing a tablet or opening a capsule will generally make its use unlicensed. Under the Medicines Act 1968, only medical and dental practitioners can customise the use of 'unlicensed' medicines. It is therefore illegal to open a capsule or crush a tablet prior to its administration without the prescriber's authorisation (preferably in writing). An alternative formulation should be found instead.

Activity 29

Complete the following table.

Medicine	Different oral formulations	Brand name
amoxicillin	capsules, oral suspension, sachets	Amoxil
furosemide		
phenytoin		
morphine sulphate		
nystatin		

Care scenario: Jack

Jack had difficulty taking his tablets, so staff decided to crush them in a mixture. One tablet was morphine sulphate modified release tablet (MST 30 mg) and Jack was given this medicine crushed in some jam. Modified release preparations are designed to release medicine at a constant rate throughout the day. However, since it was crushed, Jack received a high dose of morphine all at once and then nothing for the rest of the 12-hour period.

This resulted in his pain relief not being properly controlled and he experienced unwanted and unnecessary side effects, as he felt very sick after taking the crushed tablets and was extremely drowsy.

1. What should the staff have done instead of crushing the tablet?
2. How else could staff make sure Jack gets adequate pain relief?

Inhalation

This method is used mostly for patients who have chronic respiratory problems, such as asthma. It enables the medicine to be delivered to the site where it is most needed – the lungs. Inhalers and Nebules (for use in a nebuliser) are common examples for this route of delivery. A variety of inhalers are available on the market. Aerosols and dry powder inhalers are marketed. Compliance aids such as 'spacers', e.g. Volumatic®, can be prescribed to help with the delivery of the medicine from an inhaler.

Think about the different medicines that you give to the individuals. Do you crush any tablets to help the individual take them? Could an alternative formulation be used?

Care scenario: Steven's asthma

Steven suffers from asthma and uses a salbutamol and beclometasone inhaler. He often gets oral thrush (a fungal infection in the throat) and anti-fungal lozenges were prescribed regularly to treat it. The pharmacist advised that Steven used the salbutamol first to open the airways and then use the corticosteroid inhaler (beclometasone). Following the use of his inhalers, Steven is given a drink to rinse his mouth. A spacer (for example, a Volumatic®) was also prescribed to reduce the risk of oral thrush.

1. Why might Steven be getting oral thrush so often? (Hint: look up the side effects of his asthma medication.)
2. Do you think it is a good idea to give Steven a drink to rinse his mouth with after using the inhalers?
3. How will a spacer help reduce the risk of getting oral thrush?

Do any of the individuals in your care use an inhaler? Do you make sure that they correctly use the inhaler for maximum benefit?

Do you request compliance aids, e.g., a Volumatic ®, or alternative preparation if the individual's technique is poor? Who can advise the individual on correct inhaler use?

Injection

There are three different routes for administration by injection:

- Intramuscular injection. The medicine is injected directly into large muscles in the body, usually the legs or bottom. This can only be performed by a doctor or trained nurse.

- Intravenous injection. The medicine is administered directly into the veins. Medicines are absorbed into the body rapidly via this route, which is advantageous when a situation is life-threatening. Again, this can only be performed by a doctor or trained nurse.

- Subcutaneous injection. The medicine is administered directly in the fat layer beneath the skin. A common example is insulin.

You may, after suitable training, administer medicines via subcutaneous injection. You should be supported by policies regarding this practice. Written consent from the individual is required, and the individual's doctor and community nurse must also give permission and training.

Topically

Creams, ointments and gels are applied directly to the skin. They can be used to treat skin conditions. You may be required to apply such external preparations to individuals. Gloves should always be worn (normally latex, or latex-free gloves, if you are allergic to latex) to protect against absorption of the medication through your skin and to prevent cross-contamination.

Do you have any diabetic individuals who require regular insulin injections? What insulin do they have? What is the type of injection/system they use? Have you been trained to administer insulin? Is it within your competency?

Look in the BNF (British National Formulary) to see what different products are available to administer insulin. If you administer insulin, do you have specific protocols to follow to make sure you administer it safely? Has the individual given written consent allowing you to administer his or her insulin?

Activity 30

List all the topical preparations you have used. Record their active ingredient if they have one, and what they are prescribed for.

Cream, ointment, gel	Active ingredient	Use

Where are applications of creams recorded in the service you provide? Is it the Medicine Administration Record (MAR) chart? If not, how are cream applications recorded?

Infusion

These are when fluids and medicines are given over a period of time (for example, 12 hours) into the vein. These are usually prepared and maintained by trained nurses.

Instillation

Medicines can be instilled in the eyes, nose or ears. You may administer via this route after suitable training. Common examples include:

- ear drops for wax removal
- eye drops for the treatment of glaucoma, dry eyes or an eye infection
- nose drops or sprays to treat allergies such as hay fever, or inflammatory conditions of the nose.

All eye, ear and nose drops have an expiry date of 28 days to reduce the risk of microbial contamination – bacteria growing in the drops – which may harm the individual if instilled.

Activity 31

Write down all the eye, ear and nose drops you have used and record their use.

Eye, ear or nose drops	What are they for?

Do you record the date that the drops were opened and discard after 28 days?

TOWER HAMLETS COLLEGE
Learning Centre
Poplar High Street
LONDON
E14 0AF

Rectally

Medicines are absorbed quickly into the body by this route. Suppositories are available for this route of administration. These are inserted high into the rectum. Only suitably trained members of staff should administer medication via this route, normally on a named individual basis only. A nurse may undertake this procedure in some services instead of care staff.

Vaginally

Pessaries are formulated to be administered via this route. These are normally used to treat conditions of the vagina. You should only be administering medicines via this route if you have been suitably trained to do so. Again, a nurse may undertake this procedure in some services instead of care staff.

A common medicine administered vaginally is Clotrimazole (Canesten). This is used to treat fungal infections of the vagina which may occur, due to a course of antibiotics for example. Various formulations are available for vaginal use, for example, pessaries or a vaginal cream inserted using a special applicator.

Transdermally

The transdermal patch is becoming a more common route of administration. Examples that may be familiar to you include fentanyl patches, Hormone Replacement Therapy (HRT) patches and nicotine patches.

The drug is released slowly from the patch over a period of time and is absorbed through the skin into the bloodstream. The product information leaflet will state the most suitable sites for application and these should be rotated on a regular basis so the same site does not always have the patch applied. Normal sites are the chest, upper arms or backs of hands. The skin should be clean, dry and hair-free.

Points to remember are:

- the site of application must be varied to reduce the risk of the skin becoming sensitive to the patch, which might result in inflammation and irritation
- a record of the site used should be kept
- once the patch is removed, it should be folded in half both to prevent reapplication and to deactivate the patch.

A common example of a medicine administered rectally is rectal diazepam. It is used for the treatment of epilepsy. Have you received training to administer by this route, and is this done against a written protocol?

Have you been trained to administer all formulations that you currently do? Would further training help you? Are you able to access this? Can your manager, pharmacist or district nurse help you?

PEG (Percutaneous Endoscopic Gastrostomy) tube

Medicines may be administered via a PEG tube. All medicines should be checked with the drug company for current information on administration by this route to see what formulation is the most suitable. Drug interactions with other drugs and with food should also be considered. The community or hospital pharmacist may be able to help compile information on the best formulations to be administered. You should be suitably trained to administer medicines and you should only administer medication via this route if it is within your own competencies. Remember that written permission must be obtained from the prescriber if there are no alternative formulations and tablets have to be crushed or capsules opened (see page 44).

Activity 32

Question	Comments
Do you have any individuals in your care who require medication to be administered via a PEG tube?	
Have you compiled a list of the medicines and formulations and obtained information from the medicines' manufacturers?	
Have you recorded any advice about the most suitable formulation and any precautions that must be taken when administering via this route?	
Have you contacted the doctor if the drug manufacturer advises against giving a particular medicine via a PEG tube to obtain a different medicine or formulation? Do you feel confident to do this, or could the pharmacist help you?	
Have you been fully trained to administer medicines via this route?	
Have you obtained written permission from the prescriber if there is no alternative and the tablets have to be crushed or capsules opened?	

1. List the various formulations of medicines available on the market.

2. Where could you look for alternative formulations that may suit each individual's needs?

3. Which health care professionals may be able to help and train you to help you meet an individual's needs further?

TOWER HAMLETS COLLEGE
Learning Centre
Poplar High Street
LONDON
E14 0AF

Home remedies

Some medicines can be administered to individuals that have not been prescribed. These are usually described as home (or homely) remedies. Their administration must be supported by a home remedy policy, where each medicine is individually detailed. These are medicines that can be purchased and administered for certain clinical conditions for a maximum number of doses per day, for a maximum length of time (usually 48 hours), and any cautions or warnings must be recorded.

Their administration must be fully documented on the MAR chart together with a book recording their use with a running total recorded to make sure all doses administered are accounted for. It is normally up to the home what home remedies they buy and whether their administration is within the staff's competence to do so. It is advised that the home remedy policy is checked and signed by a clinician or pharmacist to make sure the dose and reasons to administer them are correct.

An example of a home remedy policy for the medication paracetamol is shown below.

Paracetamol 500 mg tablets	
Indication (what it is for)	For general pain, headaches, period pain
Dose	One or two tablets every four to six hours
Maximum number of doses	8 tablets in 24 hours
Maximum number of days to be administered before referral to a doctor	2 days (48 hours)
Cautions and warnings	Do not administer if already taking any product containing paracetamol

A home remedy policy for paracetamol

Activity 35

Fill in the table below.

Question	Answer
Do you have a Home Remedy Policy in your care home?	
Does it detail individual medicines or is it a list of unspecified medicines, for example, cough mixture?	
Why should individual medicines be recorded?	
What medicines could you buy to use as home remedies?	
Do you use prescribed medicines that are no longer needed? Why is it illegal to use a prescribed medicine as a home remedy?	
What would you do if relatives or friends brought medicines into the care service for administration to individuals in your care?	
Does your medication policy and the individual's contract advise what to do?	

Care scenario: Mandeep

Mandeep suffers from epilepsy and has been prescribed phenytoin. Mandeep's daughter is concerned that her father is depressed, and decides to buy some St John's wort, which is commonly purchased to treat mild depression. She does not tell the care assistants that she is giving Mandeep the herbal remedy.

Mandeep begins to have epileptic fits and the doctor is called. The doctor decides to increase the dose of phenytoin after the phenytoin levels had been taken at the hospital. Mandeep no longer has any fits and over time he becomes more settled. His daughter stops bringing in the St John's wort. Mandeep then begins to feel unwell and complains of dizziness and feeling sick. His speech becomes slurred and his eyes start to flicker. The doctor is called again and Mandeep is admitted to hospital with suspected phenytoin toxicity.

1. From reading the above account, what do you think caused Mandeep to start having epileptic fits?
2. How could the situation have been prevented?
3. What policy/policies should be put in place to prevent such an event occurring?

Activity 36

Write a home remedy policy for medicines that you might wish to purchase to use within your care service. A template has been provided below.

Name of medicine	
Indication (what it is for)	
Dose	
Maximum number of doses	
Maximum number of days to be administered before referral to a doctor	
Cautions and warnings	

Do you feel confident about administering home remedies? Is there a set protocol supporting their individual uses? Where do you record their administration?

When would you seek help from the doctor if the symptoms did not go away? Do you feel confident that friends and relatives would always discuss any medication brought into the home? Would you feel able to talk to an individual's friends and relatives if you found other medicines in the individual's room?

Safe practice in the administration of medicines

4.1 Understand the need to obtain the individual's consent (and where applicable privacy) prior to administering medicines to them

Patient consent

The following good practice must be followed before administering medicines.

- The individual must give informed consent to enable you to administer their medication to them.
- All medication prescribed must be offered to the individual but he or she has a right to refuse to take the medicines prescribed.
- The individual should not be forced to take any medicines.
- The medicines should not be hidden or disguised in food (covert administration).
- Consistent refusal to take the prescribed medication should be recorded and discussed with the doctor.

Activity 37

List reasons why an individual might refuse to take their medication.

_____

_____

_____

If an individual is unable to give informed consent to take any medication, the matter may lie with the decision made by a multidisciplinary team. They will collectively decide if it is in the person's best interest to administer medication to them or not.

This team may consist of:

- you and other care staff
- the service manager or team leader responsible for medication in the home
- the doctor
- any relatives
- the social worker
- an independent advocate (person who supports and speaks in favour of someone else).

Previous wishes of the individual must also be taken into consideration.

Care scenario: Doreen

Doreen had dementia and could not give informed consent to administer her medicines, one of which was Donepezil, prescribed by the hospital to treat her dementia. The staff decided to hide the medicine in her food. Her husband found out and complained to the manager. The problem was discussed with the doctor and he decided that it was in the best interests for Doreen to take the prescribed medication. However, her husband disagreed and did not want her to take any medication.

A multidisciplinary team meeting was held. This consisted of the doctor, husband, registered manager of the care service, Doreen's key worker in the care home and her social worker. The reasons of all the members of the team were considered and together they made a collective decision as to what was in her best interests. It was decided that all the medicines the doctor prescribed were to be administered, as it was considered to be in her best interests. The medication was to be offered and encouragement given, but if she refused it was to be hidden in her food.

1. How do you feel about the decision to hide the medication in Doreen's food if she refuses to take it?

Have you been in a situation where an individual in your care has been unable to give consent or refused to give consent? Do you think there is a difference?

Are any individuals in your care unable to give consent? Does your medication policy specify what to do in such an instance? Is the role of the multidisciplinary team discussed? Is the Mental Capacity Act observed?

Have any individuals in your care refused to give consent? If so, what did you do?

Have you ever given medicines secretly, without the individual knowing? If yes, would you do this now?

covertly
secretively

The decision to administer medicines **covertly** must never be taken lightly; it must only happen following the agreement of those involved in the individual's care and any decision must be fully documented. This decision is usually reached collectively by members of a multidisciplinary team. Medicines must never be administered covertly simply because an individual refuses to take their medication. The Mental Capacity Act 2005 must be taken into account if a person suffers from dementia, a brain injury or learning difficulties (see page 6).

At the end of this section you will understand the need to carry out a risk assessment for each individual to either self-administer their own medication or for care staff to undertake this role, and also the need for regular compliance checks to be undertaken to confirm that the individual can take their medicines as the doctor intended.

Self-administration

Self-administration is where the individual takes full responsibility to take his or her own medicine. All individuals should be encouraged to self-administer their own medication. They must be fully supported by you to ensure they do so safely. All individuals must be risk-assessed as able before they may self-administer their own medication. This should be done following a self-administration risk assessment policy.

Following the initial risk assessment, compliance checks must be undertaken to confirm that the individuals actually can self-administer their medicines safely. These must be done regularly as each individual's needs may change rapidly. It must be part of the agreement between the individual and the home that compliance checks are undertaken to confirm the individual takes the medicine as prescribed. The care service has a duty of care to make sure that any individuals who take responsibility for their own medicines do so safely.

Look at the self-administration risk assessment available in your care service. Do you risk-assess all individuals who wish to self-administer their own medicines? When do you undertake compliance checks?

Activity 38

Think about ways in which you could actually check the individual is safely taking his or her own medicines. List them below.

_____

_____

Do you understand the need to risk-assess the individual as able to self-administer their medicines? Do you understand the need to carry out compliance checks to confirm the individual can safely take the medicines as prescribed?

Do you have a self-administration risk assessment policy for your care service? If so, does it include compliance checks? Where do you record compliance checks?

At what stage would you offer more support to an individual to help him or her carry on self-administering his or her own medicines to maintain independence? What further support could be offered?

Do you know what services the local pharmacist can offer to help individuals take their medication correctly? When would you consider it unsafe for the individual to self-administer their own medicines?

How do you record compliance checks to confirm that each medication has been taken as the doctor intended? Is this recorded in the medication policy?

Compliance checks

Following a risk assessment confirming the individual can safely self-administer their own medication, you should:

- give the individual the medication and record the quantity given on the MAR chart (each individual must still have a record of all his or her prescribed medicines)
- after four or five days, calculate the number of tablets that should have been taken and how many should be left in the box
- check the actual number of tablets with the individual
- record this compliance check for each medicine on the MAR chart
- reassess if the audits show that the individual has not taken the medicine correctly and offer more support if needed to continue safe self-administration (for example, asking the pharmacist to dispense the medication in a compliance aid or prompting the individual to take the medication).

> Do not sign the MAR chart recording that you have administered the medicine yourself, since you have not. Instead you should sign and record what medicines and how many you have given to the individual to self-administer. Also, record on the MAR chart when you have checked that they have taken the medicines safely (a compliance check).

Care scenario: Kevin

Kevin was fiercely independent and wanted to self-administer his medicines. He lived at home and domiciliary care assistants visited him three times a day. He was risk-assessed as able to self-administer his tablets. His risk assessment indicated that he understood all the medicines he took and when he should take them.

Staff ordered his medication when he requested it. They did not notice that Kevin's requests for digoxin started to become far more frequent than for his other medicines. Upon visiting Kevin, one of the domiciliary care assistants found Kevin to be drowsy. Kevin also told her that he had been having diarrhoea. The care assistant put the diarrhoea down to a stomach bug that had been going around. Kevin also began to experience headaches and was regularly very tired. His health deteriorated quite rapidly and he was becoming very confused and was still very drowsy. He was admitted to hospital for observation. The hospital diagnosed digoxin toxicity. Kevin had been taking digoxin three times a day instead of daily. He had confused the digoxin with phenobarbitone as the tablets were a similar shape, colour and size. Staff had not undertaken any compliance checks at all and had failed to notice that Kevin had asked for extra supplies of digoxin too frequently.

1. How could the care assistants have prevented this? What different outcome would this have had?
2. How often should compliance checks have been undertaken?
3. What should Kevin's increased requests for prescriptions for digoxin have indicated to staff?
4. What else could have been done to stop this happening? Could the local pharmacist dispense his medication in a Monitored Dosage System? Could the care assistant have arranged this?

4.3 Understand the need for appropriate preparation prior to administering medicines

By the end of this section, you should understand basic hygiene procedures and the correct equipment and the correct documents to have before you administer any medicines.

It is important to follow basic procedures when you handle medicines:

- Employers are obliged by law to provide you with the correct equipment for any known risk you may have to deal with whilst handling medicines, in order to reduce the risk of harm to you. This may include gloves, aprons, washing facilities, spillage kits or sharps disposal containers. (See section 1.1 page 4.)

- Medicines should not be touched and extra precautions (for example, wearing gloves) must be taken for certain medicines that may cause harm if inadvertently handled. Examples of these medicines include cytotoxic medicines (medicines used to treat cancer) and application of steroid creams.

- All creams and ointments should be applied using gloves to reduce both the risk of cross-contamination and also the possibility of harm to you.

- You should always wash your hands thoroughly before starting a medicine round.

- You should never undertake a medicine round without referring to the MAR chart while you do so. This should always be referred to before the administration or application of any medicine.

- You should have current drug information readily available (see page 35 for good reference sources) to be able to confirm a dose or understand why you are administering a medicine or to check for side effects before you actually administer it.

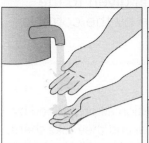

1. Wet hands with running water.

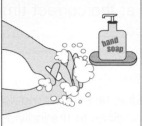

2. Rub hands together with soap and lather well, covering all surfaces.

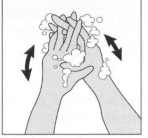

3. Weave fingers and thumbs together and slide them back and forth.

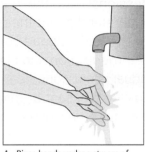

4. Rinse hands under a stream of clean, running water until all soap is gone.

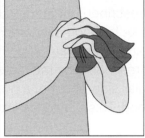

5. Blot hands dry with clean towel.

You must wash your hands properly before starting a medicine round

Activity 39

Think about your practice and then answer the following questions.

Question	Answer
Do you always wash your hands before you handle medicines?	
Do you have the relevant documents and equipment ready before you give any medicines?	
Is any extra equipment available if you need it, for example, tablet cutters, gloves?	
What would you do if you dropped a tablet on the floor?	

Look at your medication policy. Does it record the exact procedure of how to administer medicines safely?

Do you feel confident that you handle medicines in a safe and hygienic way? Do you always wear gloves to apply creams and ointments? Do you have access to medical information?

Do your MAR charts record any extra precautions that may be needed? Do you always refer to the MAR chart before the administration of any medicine and record details directly after the transaction?

Compliance is the accuracy with which an individual takes their medication as prescribed by a doctor or health professional. If you offer the medicines to the individual and they take them, they have full compliance. Individuals who self-administer their medicines should be checked regularly to make sure they have full compliance and are fully supported to achieve this.

Concordance is the shared agreement by health care professionals and the individual regarding the medication they are prescribed, what they understand about their treatment and whether they actually want to take it. Good concordance results in good compliance. You need to ensure that individuals are concordant with their medication and also are compliant in taking it. There may be reasons why the individual is not concordant. For example, they may not find a particular side effect of a medicine pleasant or may feel the medication is not doing them any good. This would lead to poor compliance (not taking his or her prescribed medication).

Following diagnosis from the clinician a prescription may be written and dispensed. Your role is to administer the medicines as the clinician has prescribed and to seek further medical help if any side effects occur.

The right individual must receive:

- the right medicine at
- the right dose at
- the right time by
- the right route.

Records of administration should record and support exactly what you have done.

Activity 40

Think about how you would demonstrate that a medicine has been administered correctly. Write down ways in which you could prove that it has.

_____

_____

Identification of the individual

You must ensure that you are giving the right medication to the right person:
- ask the individual to tell you their name
- do not prompt or say 'Are you Mrs/Mr . . . ?'

It is good practice to have other methods of identification for the individuals. You could insert an identification page in front of each individual's MAR chart. Each identification page should have a photograph of the individual, the individual's name, room number, any allergies and any special requirements. (Remember consent must be obtained before a photograph can be taken.) A template is given on page 61 as an example.

```
┌─────────────────────────────┐
│                             │
│                             │
│                             │
│         Photograph          │
│                             │
│                             │
│                             │
├─────────────────────────────┤
│ Name:                       │
│ Room number:                │
│ Allergies:                  │
│ Special requirements:       │
└─────────────────────────────┘
```

An identification page template

Care scenario: Mistaken identity

A care home looks after 26 individuals. Staff turnover is high and many agency staff come to the home to look after the individuals. There is no formal way of identifying the individuals, and agency staff often have trouble knowing who is who.

An agency care assistant who had never worked in the home before come on duty. She was told to administer the medicines since the usual care assistant was off sick. There was nobody available to help the agency care assistant with the medication round. She started the medication round and asked individuals to confirm their names before she gave them medication. All the individuals in the home responded to the names they were called, for example, 'Are you Andrew?' Later that day an individual, Joan, became very ill and the doctor was called. It was later found that Joan had received John's medication.

1. What could the agency care assistant have done to prevent this incident from occurring?
2. What documentation would also have helped to prevent this error?
3. Can you think of anything else the care assistant could have done? (Hint: think about the way the care assistant checked the individuals' names.)

Look at the medication policy for your care service. Does it enable you to administer the right medicine at the right dose to the right individual at the right time by the right route? Does it guide you through accurate recording following the transaction? What systems do you have in place to recognise the individual?

Can you identify all the individuals in your care? Think what it would be like to be new to the service. Do you think you could identify everybody who lives in the home if you were new?

Does the medication policy guide you through how to identify individuals? Do you always ask the individual's name before you administer his or her medicines if you don't know the individual very well, or do you ask him or her to confirm the name you have asked them? Which is better, and why?

Do you always refer to the MAR chart before you administer any medicines?

Controlled Drugs (CDs)

Controlled Drugs are administered in the usual way except that the administration has to be witnessed by another appropriately trained member of staff.

Activity 42

List the Controlled Drugs that you have in your care service or that you have had experience of handling.

_____

_____

_____

_____

In addition to being recorded as administered on the MAR chart, a CD also has to be recorded in the Controlled Drug Register. The person administering the CD has to record this and sign the register. The witness also has to sign the register confirming that the dose has been administered.

The quantity of CDs recorded on the MAR chart should always match the record of the running total in the CD register. In turn, these should match the actual quantity of the Controlled Drugs in the CD cabinet. It is not necessary to have two signatures on the MAR chart but it is essential to have two signatures in the CD register (the one who administered it and the one who witnessed the administration).

The CD register must record the information shown in the table on page 65. It should be a bound book with consecutive page numbers (page 1, 2, 3) so it can be easily seen if any pages have been removed. Mark in the table whether you record all this information.

Any discrepancies in the number of CDs must be reported immediately to the designated person in charge of medicines in your workplace or the registered manager. The registration authority (CSCI) must be informed. It may also be necessary to inform the police.

Information	Yes	No
The name of the individual receiving the CD.		
The drug, strength and formulation (for example, morphine sulphate 10 mg MR (modified release) tablets).		
The date and time the CD was received into the home on the page specifically for the individual and that CD. The total quantity should be recorded. This must be confirmed by counting what is in the CD cabinet.		
The date, time and quantity of the CD administered and the running balance recorded. This recorded balance (e.g. number of tablets) should be checked with the actual quantity of the CD in the CD cabinet.		
The full signature of the care assistant who administered the CD.		
The full signature of the care assistant who witnessed the transaction.		
The date and quantity of CD that is no longer required that is to be returned to the pharmacist for destruction. This may be signed by the person collecting the CD from the care home. The balance should then be zero.		

1. Do you record all Controlled Drugs on the MAR chart as well as the CD register? Are they the same?

2. Why should only one person sign the MAR chart? Does your medication policy agree with this or does it say that two people should sign the MAR chart? What is the disadvantage of two people signing the MAR chart?

3. What is the second signature recorded in the CD register for?

4. Is the balance in the CD register checked regularly with the actual quantity of CDs in the cabinet after each transaction?

5. Who do you report any missing CDs to?

Check your care home's medication policy. What does it say regarding the administration and recording of medicines? Do you feel confident that it includes all the basic points? What does it say about Controlled Drugs?

Are you confident that all the records in your care service support practice and actually record exactly what has happened? Are there any gaps in the MAR charts where someone has given a medicine but not signed it, or not given a medicine and not recorded the reason for non-administration?

Do you always refer to the MAR chart before the administration of medicines, no matter how familiar you are with the individual's medication? Do you check each labelled medicine in addition to the MAR chart to confirm it is the right medicine for that individual before you administer it?

Do the MAR charts reflect what is recorded in the CD register? Do you regularly check the quantities of CDs in the CD cabinet? If you don't, who is responsible for doing this?

4.7 Understand the requirements for careful and planned audits of medicine stock and its storage in accordance with the manufacturer's instructions and organisational policies

By the end of this section you should understand the requirements for careful and planned audits of medicine stock and their storage requirements. You should also know how to undertake audits to demonstrate that the medicines are administered as prescribed.

In domiciliary care, the requirement is to store medicines safely. Standard 10.5 National Minimum Standards for Domiciliary care requires that 'care and support staff leave medication at all times in a safe place which is known and accessible to the individual or, if not appropriate for the individual to have access, where it is only accessible to relatives and other personal carers, health personnel and domiciliary care staff'.

Storage should be at the discretion of the care staff following risk assessments. Access to medication by visitors should also be considered, for example, if small children visit the individual.

The manager or designated staff for all services are normally responsible for auditing medicines to confirm that medicines have been administered as prescribed. All quantities of medicines received should be recorded to enable general audits to be undertaken. In addition,

Activity 45

Complete the following table to reflect on the storage of medicine in your care service.

Question	What happens in your care service?
Are all medicines stored in a clean, lockable facility?	
Do you use a medicine trolley? Is it big enough?	
Are trolleys secured to a wall when not in use?	
All medicine must be stored at a temperature below 25° C at all times. Are yours? How could this be achieved if not?	
Medicines may require refrigeration. The maximum, minimum and current refrigerator temperature should be recorded on a daily basis and the temperature should lie between 2° C and 8° C at all times. Does yours? What do you do if temperatures fall outside the limits?	
Is it a designated medication refrigerator or do you use the food refrigerator? If so, are medicines securely stored within?	
Controlled Drugs (CD) must be stored in cupboards that comply with the Misuse of Drugs (Safe Custody) Regulations (1973), as amended. Controlled Drug cabinets should be reserved for CDs only. Items such as jewellery, money or cigarettes should not be stored in a CD cabinet. Do you have a CD cabinet? Does it comply with the regulations? If so, does it hold CDs only?	
Access to medication should be limited. For each shift there should be a designated person to hold the keys for all medication cabinets, trolleys and refrigerators. Is there a designated person who holds the keys in your care service?	

staff should be monitored to confirm that they do actually administer the medicines and record the transaction. Audits should be undertaken as frequently as necessary, normally a minimum of monthly. If, for example, the general audits show that many mistakes are made, they should be done more frequently before and after a medication round to identify which care assistant is responsible for the incorrect administration or poor recording of medicines. Support and further training can then be offered to improve practice.

Activity 46

Question	Answer
Where are the medicines stored? Are all medicines held in a locked cabinet or trolley at all times or safely in someone's own home?	
Do you consider storage in your care service to be safe?	
How could it be improved?	
In a care home, what would you do in the event of an emergency? Do you feel that medicines would still be safely stored if you were distracted by an emergency whilst you were giving out the medicines?	

Care scenario: David

David lives at home but receives domiciliary care three times a day for personal care and help administering his medicines. He has grown-up children who visit on a regular basis. David has always left his medicines on his bedside cabinet. One day staff noticed that some tablets were missing from a blister pack in his bedroom. David said he had not taken the tablets but mentioned that a young grandchild had visited the night before and had played for a while in his bedroom while David was talking to his daughter.

1. What can the care assistant do to find out how many tablets have been removed from the blister pack?
2. What can be done to avoid this happening again?

Do you have good auditing systems within your care service? Are these undertaken regularly, at least once a month? Can you tell instantly if medicines have not been administered, or if they are missing?

Do you store all medicines correctly in your care service? Are external medicines separate from internal medicines? What do you do with each new 28-day supply of medicines received? Are these locked away if they are not used immediately?

Do you lock away medicines that are awaiting return to the pharmacy or clinical waste company for destruction? Do you feel confident that all medicines are stored at the correct temperature (so they don't deteriorate or degrade)?

What auditing system do you have in your care service? Can it identify individual staff who may not administer medicines correctly or record what they have done accurately?

CONGRATULATIONS – you have almost finished this training book. It should have improved your knowledge and understanding of handling medicines in social care.

This final section will encourage you to reflect on what you have learned from the whole course, and should encourage you to think about your practice and to improve practice, supported by your policies and procedures.

Go back to section 1.1, page 7, and answer the questions there again. Has your opinion changed? Now complete the following table below.

Question	Answer
Do you think you have met the National Minimum Standards and outcomes now that you have completed the course?	
Has your opinion changed?	
If it has, why?	
Read the section for medication on the inspection report again. Has your original opinion changed?	
Do you think now that it accurately reflects the practice in your care service?	
What could you do to improve practice further?	

Go back to section 1.1, Activity 7 (page 10). Complete the table there and then complete the table below.

Question	Answer
Overall, do you think you follow the good practice for each section in the guidance documents?	
How could you make improvements to your service?	

Go back to section 1.2, page 13.

Question	Answer
What do you think of your medication policy now?	
How would you improve it?	

Trainer notes

These Trainer notes have been written to help you give the best advice and guidance possible to your care workers. A selection of the activities on pages 2–73 are discussed, along with further ways in which you can encourage successful completion of training. The Trainer notes will also give you guidance on what additional texts or information sources you will need to give trainees opportunities to achieve the most from this book.

1. Legislation and medication

1.1 Be aware of the legislation and guidance that controls the prescribing, dispensing, administration, storage and disposal of medicines

This section (pages 2–13) will guide you through the relevant acts, regulations and guidance documents that control and support good practice in all aspects of medicine management. Staff and individuals are protected by these regulations and acts and should be aware of them. You will need to find the relevant National Minimum Standards (NMS) for the service you provide. Your staff should understand the detail and the outcomes that are expected of them in order to provide good care.

Activity 1

Before trainees fill in the table, encourage them to think about why acts and regulations exist and how they protect staff and individuals in their care alike.

Activity 2

Encourage trainees to think of medicines they handle that may require extra precautions. Examples might include cytotoxic medicines, creams and ointments, and tablets that may need crushing if an alternative cannot be found. Encourage trainees to think about why legislation exists. Trainees should identify that legislation exists to protect themselves, the individuals in their care and the general public.

Care scenario: The 'strawberry milkshake'

1. The care home can be prosecuted under the Health and Safety at Work Act (1974).

2. The situation could have been avoided by making sure proper containers for cleaning fluids are used and clearly labelled. In addition, cleaning fluids should always be stored securely, even when in use, and locked away when no longer being used.

Activity 3

This activity could be performed as a group activity prior to completion of the table. Obtain some product information/data sheets for COSHH substances in your service. Ask trainees to look at them and discuss what they would do if an accident occurred involving one of the substances. Get trainees to discuss where they think the best place to store this information is.

Activity 4

You can download the National Minimum Standards for care services from the Commission for Social Care Inspection website. A link to this site is available at www.heinemann.co.uk/hotlinks – just enter the express code 2315P. In addition to looking at the Standards for your service, trainees could also be asked to look at the Standards for other care providers. Ask trainees to comment on themes that are common to standards, as well as differences between them.

Activity 5

You will need to provide trainees with a copy of the latest CSCI inspection report, which includes the inspection for medication. Ask trainees to read the report and discuss whether or not they agree with its contents.

Activity 6

When completing this activity, trainees should be encouraged to discuss the best way and place to store medical records, including MAR charts. Do they think it is acceptable to keep records on top of the medicine trolley in an entrance hall, or do they think they should be kept in a place not accessible to general staff and visitors?

Care scenario: The handyman

1. Yes, the care home has broken the law by not protecting the information it holds about its residents.
2. The handyman broke the Access to Health and Records Act (1990) by accessing someone's medical history and then discussing it without their consent.

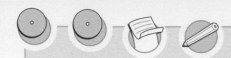

Activity 7

This activity can be a group activity. Provide trainees with a copy of the Administration and Control of Medicines in Care Homes and Children's Services guidance document. This can be accessed by visiting the Royal Pharmaceutical Society of Great Britain website – a link to this site can be found at www.heinemann.co.uk/hotlinks. Enter the express code 2315P. This is quite a lengthy document and should be given to trainees well in advance. It is also recommended that you break the document down into the main subject headings. Duplicate the table in the activity on to a flip chart and ask the group their thoughts about their current practice and whether they think it is best practice. Do they think any improvements could be made? This exercise can be repeated after the course to identify changes in opinion and practice.

Activity 8

This activity gives trainees an opportunity to consolidate their knowledge regarding legislation and explore ways to improve practice by identifying shortfalls.

1.2 Understand the legal framework and how the organisation's policies and procedures reflect these, for safe handling of medicines (prescribing, dispensing, administration, storage and disposal) by all care workers

Care scenario: The medicine mix-up

1. The serious harm caused to the individual could have been prevented if the care home's medication policy included guidance on what to do in this situation. A good policy would have advised the care assistant to seek immediate medical help and not wait until the manager came on duty.

Activity 9

Provide trainees with a copy of medication policies. Duplicate the table on page 13 and use it to encourage group discussion, completing it as you go.

2. Roles, responsibilities and boundaries

2.1 Understand the process by which medicines are prescribed, dispensed and obtained by the individual and the worker's role in the process

This section (pages 14–39) will help trainees understand the roles, responsibilities and boundaries of all workers with regard to the safe handling of medicines within various areas of care, for example, care homes (with or without nursing), day services, an individual's own home, sheltered accommodation, supported living, and other networks and services. Your service will probably only deal with one aspect of care but it is important to see what standards other care providers have to maintain.

In order to help trainees achieve this learning outcome, it is helpful if you provide them with a list of all the staff in your care service as well as their job title. This can be used as a basis for discussion and will help trainees understand everyone's roles and boundaries. Trainees should also complete Activity 10 on page 15.

Care scenario: Staff shortages

1. The domiciliary care agency received a Statutory Requirement Notice because the clerical assistant carried out duties for which she was not trained.

2. The agency could have prevented this situation from happening by making adequate arrangements in the event of a staff shortage.

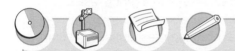

Activity 10

This activity is designed to encourage trainees to think about who is responsible for the variety of tasks involved with medicine management in their care service.

2.2 Understand the roles and boundaries of all workers with regard to the safe handling of medicines (prescribing, dispensing, administration, storage and disposal) in various care contexts

Activity 11

This activity is designed to encourage trainees to think about their own work practice and whether they feel it is within their competencies.

Activity 12

This activity encourages trainees to think about their practice and where legislation fits into this. You should be prepared to seek further training if trainees feel they need it.

2.3 Understand the need to check that the medicine received matches the medication and dosage prescribed by the clinician and is listed on the appropriate documentation

Activity 13

This activity asks the trainee to look closely at a prescription, something they may never have done. Obtain some prescriptions (or copies) for trainees to look at and ask them to identify the type of information that is common to each.

As an additional activity, give each trainee a blank prescription (a mock prescription is available on page 99 and at www.heinemann.co.uk/hotlinks – just enter the express code 2315P) and ask trainees to fill in the following details:

- their own name, address and date of birth
- 15 amoxicillin 250 mg (one, three times a day)
- 28 furosemide 20 mg (one each morning)
- 20 zopiclone 3.75 mg (one at night as required).

This exercise will help trainees to check prescriptions for errors before they are dispensed as they will develop a better understanding of what information should be included and what omissions/errors to look for.

Care scenario: Joe

1. The care assistant could have avoided this situation by checking the prescription for a signature when she picked it up from the surgery. She could have then asked for the prescription to be signed before leaving the surgery.

2. The care service could have explored other ways of collecting prescriptions and the dispensed medications for the people in their care. For example, the pharmacy may offer a collection and delivery service to avoid care assistants having to pick up prescriptions.

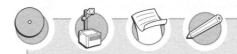

Activity 15

Either individually or in a group, ask trainees to think about the process involved in ordering prescriptions in your care service. If working in a group, the table on pages 21–22 can be used as a prompt and answers can be written on a flip chart or OHP. Ask trainees to consider whether or not they think their procedures reflect good practice. This exercise can be used as an opportunity to fill in any gaps in your medication policy to improve practice in the service.

Care scenario: Once or twice a day?

1. The home should have checked the prescription before dispensing and if accurate made a photocopy of it so that, in the event of confusion, they could check what the correct dose was.

2. A photocopy of the prescription should be kept alongside the MAR chart so that it becomes a working document. This makes the process of checking the actual dose a lot easier. A mistake that is not noticed immediately may be noticed later and corrected.

3. It is important to reduce the risk of harm to individuals through proper checking procedures.

Care scenario: Running out of medication

1. Staff could have avoided this situation by making sure they recognise if there are insufficient quantities of medication to last the cycle. If quantities are found to be insufficient, the issue can be addressed with the doctor before the medication is dispensed.

2. To avoid this happening again, staff should inform the surgery so that the surgery's records can be changed to the correct quantity to last the 28-day cycle.

Care scenario: Jane

1. The first care assistant should have recorded the doctor's verbal instructions in the daily records and insisted that the doctor wrote the full directions on the prescription.

2. The second care assistant should have contacted the doctor immediately to check the dose.

3. The MAR chart should have been referred to before any of Jane's medicines were administered.

4. It should have been noted in the MAR chart that the antibiotic was not in the MDS.

5. Staff may forget to administer medicines not in the Monitored Dosage System (MDS). To combat this, it can be highlighted on the MAR chart that the medicines are not in the MDS but in a box in the trolley. Alternatively, a card can be inserted in the MDS indicating that an extra medicine not in the MDS is to be administered (or both).

Activity 16

Ask trainees to think about any problems they have encountered when ordering prescriptions. Encourage them to identify the reasons for these problems along with practical solutions. For example, if prescriptions are not received on time each month, a meeting could be set up with the practice manager to discuss the problem. If a trainee has experienced running out of medicines, it may be because they have failed to identify that not enough medicine was prescribed in the first place.

Activity 17

You will need to gather together some medicines for the trainees to look at. You could use medicines that are no longer needed and are awaiting collection from the pharmacist.

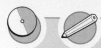

Activity 18

Gather some old MAR charts for trainees to look at. Try to include both handwritten and pharmacist-printed MAR charts. Trainees are asked to complete the MAR chart on page 98, although you may prefer them to complete a blank MAR chart that your service uses.

Care scenario: Peter

1. No, the MAR chart no longer recorded a complete record of Peter's drug regime as specified in the Care Home Regulations 2001.

2. The staff should have recorded the 'carry over' balance on the MAR chart and recorded when the next dose was due. This would highlight when Peter should receive his injection.

3. Staff should contact the health clinic if the district nurse fails to show up.

Care scenario: Eric

1. If a member of staff had written the MAR chart correctly with the right dose and quantities and removed the warfarin strengths that are not needed from the trolley, the risk of error would have been reduced.

2. The confusion over Eric's medication may have been responsible for any instability in his blood test results and subsequent changes in his dosage of warfarin.

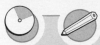

Activity 19

Trainees can complete the blank MAR chart on page 98 or, if you prefer, they can complete a MAR chart used in your service. The MAR chart on page 98 shows how it should be completed.

Care scenario: Freadah

1. If the care service had a system in place for checking prescriptions against MAR charts before administering medication, the correct dose would have been identified and the situation prevented.

Activity 20

Encourage trainees to think about the consequences that might occur if they fail to check a new individual's drug regime. Trainees should be asked what they would do if medicine labels are altered, dates are old or if they are unable to anticipate whether or not they will run out of a medicine before the next 28-day delivery.

Care scenario: Mohammed

1. Staff should have checked Mohammed's current medication regime with the doctor at the earliest opportunity to ensure they had all of Mohammed's medication. The care home could then get a supply of the epilepsy medication and administer it to Mohammed.

MEDICATION ADMINISTRATION RECORD SHEETS

NAME	ERIC SMITH		D.O.B.	3 / 1 / 12
ALLERGIES	NONE KNOWN		DOCTOR	Love
ADDRESS	The Care Home			
START DATE	1 / 3 /06	PERIOD 1 / 3 /06 ---> 28 /3 /06	START DAY	Wednesday

MEDICATION DETAILS	COMMENCING DATE	WEEK 1							WEEK 2							WEEK 3							WEEK 4						
		1	2	3	4	5	6	7	8	9	10	11	12	13	14	15	16	17	18	19	20	21	22	23	24	25	26	27	28
	HOUR : DOSE	W	T	F	S	S	M	T	W	T	F	S	S	M	T	W	T	F	S	S	M	T	W	T	F	S	S	M	T
WARFARIN 1mg Tabs — Two to be taken on alternate days	M / N / T 2 / B	X 〈2〉 T X 〈2〉 T X 〈2〉 M X 〈2〉 M X — X — X — X — X — X — X																											
received 1 / 3 /06 quant. 56 by D.M	returned quant. by destroyed quant. by																												
WARFARIN 3mg Tabs — One to be taken on alternate days	M / N / T 1 / B	T 〈1〉 X 〈1〉 T 〈1〉 X 〈1〉 M X M X — X — X — X — X — X — X																											
received 1 / 3 /06 quant. 56 by D.M	returned quant. by destroyed quant. by																												
WARFARIN 1mg Tabs — Two to be taken Saturdays & Sundays	M / N / T 2 / B	X X 〈2〉〈2〉 X X X X 〈2〉〈2〉 X X X X 〈2〉〈2〉 X X																											
received 9 / 3 /06 quant. +48 by M.D	returned quant. by destroyed quant. by																												
WARFARIN 3mg Tabs — One to be taken Mondays to Fridays	M / N / T 1 / B	X X 〈1〉〈1〉〈1〉〈1〉〈1〉 X X 〈1〉〈1〉〈1〉〈1〉〈1〉 X X 〈1〉〈1〉																											
received 9 / 3 /06 quant. +52 by M.D	returned quant. by destroyed quant. by																												
	M / N / T / B																												
received quant. by	returned quant. by destroyed quant. by																												
	M / N / T / B																												
received quant. by	returned quant. by destroyed quant. by																												

A - refused   B - nausea or vomiting   C - hospitalised   D - social leave   E - refused & destroyed

F - other (define)

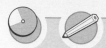

Activity 21

Trainees should create a template that includes the following:

- name of person who received the verbal information
- name of doctor or surgery staff member
- date and time
- medicines the individual brought into the home or the drug regime the individual is following
- any alternation in the drug regime
- prescriptions requested and the name of who is to collect
- a check that the information was repeated back to the doctor or surgery staff.

Care scenario: Jonathan

1. Verbal instructions regarding medication should be taken by trained staff only.

2. Verbal instructions must be recorded on a proper template, which will prompt questions that make sure all the necessary information is taken down. The verbal instructions should be repeated back, which will confirm that they have been taken down correctly.

3. The accuracy of verbal instructions can be checked by requesting that a written copy of the instructions is sent to the care service as soon as possible, preferably by fax.

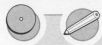

Activity 22

An additional activity could be performed with a group of trainees using role play. One trainee can play the part of the doctor and read out a prescription to another trainee, who should record what is said. This should demonstrate how easy it is to write things down inaccurately. Check whether or not the trainee recording the information repeats back the instructions. Trainees can then create a template and repeat this activity.

2.4 Understand the need to seek guidance and support (and from where) about the medicine and dosage prescribed for any particular individual

Activity 24

Trainees should be supplied with the PILs for atenolol, furosemide, aspirin and amoxicillin. Your pharmacist may be able to help you acquire these. Trainees should also have access to the BNF.

Atenolol and furosemide can in rare instances cause a rash, but the individual has been taking these medicines for a while, so they are unlikely to be the cause. There are no reports of aspirin causing rashes and, although possible, it is also unlikely to be the cause. The rash had a sudden onset and coincided with the individual taking the antibiotic amoxicillin. A rash is a common side effect of this medication.

(continued)

Activity 24 (*continued*)

The pharmacist could be contacted for advice if staff feel unsure why an adverse reaction has occurred. The doctor must be informed and they will decide what to do. If the rash occurs out of hours and both the pharmacy and the doctor's surgery are closed, staff could telephone NHS Direct for advice. The trainee must document and follow any verbal instructions given by the doctor.

Care scenario: Mrs Ghuman's crocodile

1. Along with nausea, constipation, dizziness and headaches, the side effects of Tramadol also include hallucinations.

2. The care staff should inform the doctor of Mrs Ghuman's hallucinations. The doctor will then prescribe an alternative form of pain relief.

Activity 25

You will need to give each trainee an old MAR chart and ask them to look up the side effects of the medicines listed. Trainees should document all the possible side effects and use their knowledge of the individual, in conjunction with their daily records, to assess whether or not the individual experiences any of the side effects. Ask trainees to consider whether the side effects are acceptable or not. Be prepared to take appropriate action if side effects are identified as affecting an individual's quality of life.

2.5 Understand the need for confidentiality, when and to whom information about an individual's medication may be disclosed or discussed

Trainees need to understand the need for confidentiality, when and to whom information about an individual's medication may be disclosed or discussed. For example, information may be discussed with a doctor, pharmacist and other care professionals. However, consent will be needed to discuss information with relatives or a solicitor with enduring power of attorney. You should be familiar with the two acts that relate directly to patient confidentiality, which are the Access to Health Records Act 1990 and the Data Protection Act 1998.

Discuss with trainees scenarios within your care service where staff may have been tempted to, or actually did, breach one of the above acts. Ask trainees to think how similar events could be avoided. A role-play method of exploring this will also teach trainees how and how not to act in such situations. Activity 26 on page 39 and the Care scenario on page 38 could be used in role-play exercises.

Ask trainees to imagine a situation where a colleague read their private medical notes. Help the trainees discuss their feelings about this and ask them what the possible outcomes might be (for example, any harm or damage). Next, ask the trainees to imagine a situation where they have access to someone else's medical file. What harm could potentially come of this, especially if they discovered something significant, for example, that a Catholic patient had once had an abortion? Discuss with the trainees ways of preventing access to medical records in your care service.

Care scenario: The notice board

1. The children's home broke the Access to Health Records Act 1990 and the Data Protection Act 1998. This could result in possible prosecution of the children's home.

2. Both the aunt and her niece suffered as a consequence of this event. The aunt was upset because she assumed that as her 15-year-old niece was taking the contraceptive pill, she must be sexually active. The niece was also affected by this event because her confidential records should not be accessible to anyone without her consent.

Activity 26

The trainee should thank Vera's daughter for bringing the matter to their attention but say that they cannot discuss what medicine Vera is currently taking unless Vera has previously given consent. If she hasn't, the trainee should reassure Vera's daughter that they will observe Vera and discuss any change in her condition with the doctor, consultant or prescribing nurse. It is important that the trainee knows that they cannot discuss any medical condition without prior consent from the individual in their care.

When Vera asks what medication she is taking, the trainee should understand that they are able to tell her. Under the Access to Health Records Act and the Data Protection Act, individuals have a legal right to know what has been written in their files or recorded anywhere else. Trainees should talk with Vera about how she feels and investigate further the reasons why she feels unwell. This may be a direct side effect of the medicine

she has recently been prescribed. Any relevant information gained from talking with Vera should be discussed with the doctor and an alternative medication may be prescribed.

3. Types of medicine and routes of administration

3.1 Understand the importance of some types of medication prescribed and administered to individuals

This section (pages 40–53) focuses on the different formulations of medicines available and their routes of delivery. It also looks at common side effects and adverse reactions, as well as reasons why some medicines should not be given together. Trainees need to be familiar with all the medicines they administer and what they are given for. Access to information about medicines is important, and recognising side effects and common doses is essential for good care of individuals.

Care scenario: Kathleen

1. Kathleen was regularly having diarrhoea because each of the three medicines she was being given are for constipation. The diarrhoea was caused by administering all three laxatives together. They were also still administered once the diarrhoea cleared up. Kathleen was probably not suffering

from constipation. Had the care assistants known what the medicines were for, they would have questioned the drug regime and asked the doctor to review Kathleen's medication. Finally, the care assistants did not give the Movicol correctly. This medicine was prescribed to be given when required and not routinely.

Activity 27

This activity helps trainees learn about the importance of some commonly prescribed medicines, as well as their common adult doses and possible side effects.

3.2 Understand the classification of medicine

Activity 28

You will need to gather together at least five different medicines. Most medicines are dispensed in their generic form (e.g. salbutamol) but the pharmacist may supply branded formulations (e.g. Ventolin®) and label them generically. Try to select examples of this. Ask trainees to look carefully at the box to see if they have 'POM' or 'P' printed on them. You cannot buy a POM over the counter but you can buy a P medicine. Paracetamol is a good example: a box of 16 tablets is a GSL medicine, a box of 32 tablets is a P medicine and a box of 100 tablets is a POM. Trainees will need the Controlled Drug register to identify CDs.

3.3 Understand the different routes by which medicines are administered and by whom

Trainees need to understand that medicines can be administered by a variety of routes. They need to be aware of the different routes and should know whether or not they are competent/allowed to administer medicines by certain routes.

Care scenario: Jack

1. Staff should have thought about using a different formulation that may be more appropriate for Jack.

2. Staff could ask the doctor for an alternative form of the medication such as a liquid preparation or a transdermal patch.

Care scenario: Steven's asthma

1. The corticosteroid inhaler (beclometasone) can cause oral thrush as a side effect.

2. Taking a drink after using a steroid inhaler is advised. This is because rinsing the mouth may help prevent oral thrush as it washes the steroid from the throat.

3. A spacer will help reduce the risk of oral thrush by reducing the speed of the aerosol particles and their impact in the throat. A spacer also allows more time for the particles to be inhaled and deposited in the lungs, preventing them from being left at the back of the throat.

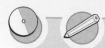

Activity 31

You may like to gather together some eye, ear and nose drops and look at them with a group of trainees. Try to include some drops that need to be discarded after 28 days so that trainees can see if the date of opening was recorded. This is a good opportunity to reflect on current practice in your service. Do all drops have to be stored in a refrigerator? Are all drops stored correctly? The storage instructions are usually found in the PIL, on the box or on the pharmacist label.

Activity 32

The PEG method of drug administration is very specialist and training should be sought from a healthcare professional. It is important for trainees to think about the medicines they may give via a PEG. Ask trainees if they crush tablets or open capsules. Encourage them to think about alternative formulations, drug-drug interactions and drug-food interactions.

3.4 Understand the importance of noting and reporting any changes to individuals following administration of medicine

Activity 33

The most likely reason for Anna's red rash and swollen hands is flucloxacillin. The doctor must be informed immediately of the reaction and care plans should record exactly what happened and any actions taken. In order to prevent the situation from happening again, the MAR chart and care plans must record that Anna is allergic to flucloxacillin. The pharmacist must also be informed so that they can update their records.

Care scenario: Gideon

1. A possible side effect of Enalapril is a persistent dry cough.

2. Instead of buying Gideon some cough and sore throat remedies, staff should have first checked to see if a cough is a side effect of Gideon's medication. Staff should have then made Gideon an appointment to see the doctor, who would make the link between the Enalapril and Gideon's sore throat. The doctor would then prescribe Gideon an alternative medication.

Activity 34

You may want to gather a collection of MAR charts. For any individuals who do have allergies, gather the last twelve months of MAR charts and ask trainees to see if the allergies have been routinely recorded on each MAR chart.

3.5 Understand the need to check contra indications and medicine interactions prior to administration of home remedies or over-the-counter medicines, and complementary medicines and preparations

Activity 35

If you have a home remedy policy, ensure all trainees have been given a copy. Discuss in a group whether it contains all the information that is necessary to safely administer home remedies or over-the-counter medicines (use the example of paracetamol on page 52 to compare). Ask the trainees where they record the administration of home remedies and what audit system is used to keep account of the home remedies on the premises.

Care scenario: Mandeep

1. It is almost certain that Mandeep began having epileptic fits because of the St John's wort he was taking.

2. Mandeep's daughter should have told staff that she was giving Mandeep a herbal remedy.

3. To help prevent this type of situation happening again, the care service needs to put in place a policy that requires all medicines brought into the home to be given to staff. Staff can then check for possible drug interactions before administering them. Friends and relatives of individuals in the home should be encouraged to discuss any requests to bring alternative therapies into the home before they do so. The policy could be included in the contract between the individual and the care service.

Activity 36

Encourage trainees to write a home remedy policy. Gather some examples of home remedies and ask trainees to choose one to create a policy for. They should be able to complete this activity using the table on page 53 and the PIL supplied with the home remedy. In practice, it is advisable to ask a pharmacist or doctor to check the policy for accuracy before it is implemented.

4. Safe practice in the administration of medicines

4.1 Understand the need to obtain the individual's consent (and where applicable privacy) prior to administering medicines to them

This section (pages 54–73) covers the safe practice in the administration of medicines and includes accurate record keeping. Patient consent and self-administration are also discussed.

Activity 37

Ask trainees to write down reasons why individuals might refuse medication. It may be helpful to first explore reasons why they themselves have not taken medication prescribed to them. For example, do they always finish a course of antibiotics and if not, why not?

Care scenario: Doreen

1. This Care scenario gives trainees the opportunity to explore their thoughts and feelings about the decision to administer Doreen's medication without her consent. Encourage them to put themselves in Doreen's position and then in Doreen's husband's position. Does their opinion change? Discuss hiding medicines in food (covert administration) and ask whether they think this is ever acceptable. Again, encourage trainees to think how they would feel if the person being given medication secretively was them. You should also explore the Mental Capacity Act 2005 with trainees here.

4.2 Understand the need to carry out a risk assessment for each individual requiring medication

Activity 38

Trainees should realise that individuals may pass a risk assessment to safely self-administer medicine, but they may not actually take their medicines. This may be because of a refusal to take the medicine or because they have forgotten. Trainees should identify that they could check whether or not an individual is taking their medicines by:

- giving the individual a set amount of medicine and then checking the amount of medicine left after a few days (e.g. number of tablets)

- removing all medicines at the end of each month and identifying why there are any remaining if a 28-day supply was provided

- encouraging cleaning staff to report any medicines they find during routine cleaning of the individual's room.

Care scenario: Kevin

1. The care assistants could have prevented this situation by carrying out compliance checks. Kevin's mix-up with his medication would therefore have been picked up very quickly.

2. Compliance checks should have been carried out after the first five days and at the end of each 28-day cycle.

3. Kevin's more frequent requests for digoxin should have alerted staff to the fact that Kevin was running out of this medication too quickly.

4. Had the domiciliary care assistant known about the possible side effects of Kevin's medication, they may have been alerted to the possibility that he wasn't taking it correctly. The pharmacist could have supplied Kevin's medication in an MDS and the care assistant could have arranged this.

4.3 Understand the need for appropriate preparation prior to administering medicines

Failure to prepare before the administration of medicines may lead to drug administration errors.

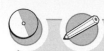

Activity 39

Encourage trainees to think carefully about their practice. Are they supplied with all the necessary equipment to successfully undertake their duties? Is their practice supported by the service's medication policy? In addition to this activity, you could obtain leaflets detailing how to wash hands properly or use the illustrations on page 59, using them as a discussion tool. To make the activity more participatory, you can also gather together all the items needed to safely and successfully administer medicines (for example, a MAR chart, a pen, an identification page, a tablet cutter, medicine tots, a jug of water, cups, a tablet counter, etc.).

4.4 Understand the need to ensure that the correct dose, of the correct medication, is given to the correct person at the correct time by the correct route or method

Activity 40

As an additional activity, give trainees some old MAR charts and ask them to identify how they prove a medicine has been administered correctly. Have the following been recorded?

- The name of the individual.
- The start date of the MAR chart.

- The medicine name, dose, formulation and directions, and time of administration.
- Two signatures to say that the medicine has been checked.

Also ask trainees to consider if all medicines were accurately checked in, whether or not there was a copy of the prescription to check against, if there are any gaps on the MAR chart and if any reasons are given for non-administration. Does the balance of medicines left tally with the total in the returns book?

Care scenario: Mistaken identity

1. The agency care assistant should have asked for a permanent member of the home's staff to be with her during the medication round. The permanent member of staff could have helped correctly identify individuals.

2. Alongside the MAR chart, a facing sheet with a photograph of the individual would help the agency care assistant prevent the error.

3. The care assistant could have asked people their name instead of asking if they were a particular person, i.e. 'What's your name please?' instead of 'Are you Andrew?'

4.5 Understand the need to record correctly the medication given, to whom the medication is given, the time and dosage at which it is given, the method of administration, and comments and signature after each administration

Are staff audited before and after a medicine round to demonstrate that they actually do administer medicines correctly and accurately record what they have done? Is this something that could be introduced? You will need to decide how often this could be done (i.e. in line with eight-weekly supervision or more/less frequently?). A staff drug audit chart can be downloaded by visiting www.heinemann.co.uk/hotlinks – just enter the express code 2315P.

Activity 41

The use of role play may be helpful with this activity. Ask the trainees to pretend to administer a medicine (sweets can be used as a substitute) and record what they have done on a MAR chart. Afterwards, ask other trainees:

- Was the individual receiving the medicine identified?
- Did the trainee look at the MAR chart before administering the medicine?
- Did the trainee check the medicine before administering it?
- Did the trainee read the label as well as the MAR chart?
- Was the medicine offered to the individual?
- Was the event properly recorded?
- If the medicine was not administered, was this recorded?

Care scenario: Bill's double dose

1. Yes, this was a preventable error.
2. The first care assistant should have recorded the administration of Bill's medication immediately after it was given.

Activity 42

It is advisable that trainees create their list of Controlled Drugs by using old empty boxes. Ask trainees to look at the CD register and identify any instances of crossing out, missing signatures and incorrect balances. In addition, ask trainees to look at the dates of administration and identify any that are missing. Do the entries on the CD register match with what is recorded on the MAR charts?

4.6 Understand the need to report and seek advice

Many errors made in medicine administration are common. If the reasons for the error are identified, the risk of repeating the error is reduced. You may wish to ask a trainee if they have ever made any errors. Ask them why they think the error occurred and how it could have been prevented.

Activity 43

This could become a group activity, with trainees thinking of reasons why the errors occurred and ways to prevent them. Ask the group if their service's medication policy supports good practice in such a way as to prevent the errors occurring.

Care scenario: The interruption

1. The care assistant should have reported the mistake straight away and not waited until Paul became ill.

2. Paul's next of kin should have been informed immediately. The next of kin would almost certainly want to be with Paul while he was in hospital and, had Paul died, his next of kin would not have been able to be with him during his final hours.

3. The care home needs to investigate the reasons for the mistake and make sure that staff carrying out medication rounds are not interrupted. The home's medication policy will have to be rewritten to reflect this improvement in practice.

4.7 Understand the requirements for careful and planned audits of medicine stock and its storage in accordance with the manufacturer's instructions and organisational policies

Activity 45

This activity focuses on the safe storage of medicines. Trainees should be able to assess whether storage in your care service is adequate and in line with the NMS. Be prepared to improve any storage requirements necessary to improve your practice.

Care scenario: David

1. The care assistant can count the tablets left in the blister pack and check this against how many tablets have been recorded as received and administered.

2. A risk assessment should be carried out, which should identify the need to store David's medication in a more secure location.

4.8 Understand the need for the prompt and safe disposal of unwanted or out-of-date medicines

Care scenario: Medicine disposal

1. Access to the room should be restricted to staff members responsible for medication only. In addition, all medicines in the room should be locked in a cabinet.

Activity 47

You can use this activity to also encourage trainees to think about the following questions.

- Are unwanted medicines removed from the medicine trolley?

- Where are unwanted medicines stored?

- Are unwanted medicines locked away or left in an open box for collection?

- Are these medicines recorded in a 'returns book'?

- Is the audit trail for unwanted medicines always completed?

Student log

The following tables have been reproduced with the kind permission of Skills for Care. Use these tables to log your progress during your training and record the learning outcomes you have covered. The tables may also be used to map the content of an NVQ qualification or other relevant training course. For full details of how the knowledge set for medication cross-references NVQ units, Common Induction Standards and GSCC Code of Practice (workers), please see the Skills for Care knowledge set document. A link to the documents on the skillsforcare.org.uk website has been made available at www.heinemann.co.uk/hotlinks. Simply enter the express code 2315P when you access the site.

Main area	Learning outcome	Learning outcome achieved (manager's or trainer's signature)	Date
1. Legislation and medication	1.1 Be aware of the legislation and guidance that controls the prescribing, dispensing, administration, storage and disposal of medicines: ■ Medicines Act 1968 + amendments ■ Misuse of Drugs Act 1971 (Controlled Drugs) + amendments ■ Health and Safety at Work Act 1974 ■ COSHH Regulations 1999 ■ Care Standards Act 2000 (Receipt, storage and administration of medicines) ■ Access to Health Records Act 1990 ■ Data Protection Act 1998 ■ Hazardous Waste Regulations 2005 ■ Administration and Control of Medicines in Care Homes and Children's Services (June 2003)		
	1.2 Understand the legal framework, and how the organisation's policies and procedures reflect these, for safe handling of medicines (prescribing, dispensing, administration, storage and disposal) by all workers.		

Main area	Learning outcome	Learning outcome achieved (manager's or trainer's signature)	Date
2.1 Roles, responsibilities and boundaries	2.1 Understand the process by which medicines are prescribed, dispensed and obtained by the individual and the worker's role in this process: ■ Prescribers (medical and non-medical) ■ Managers ■ Social care staff ■ Ancillary staff ■ Clerical staff/administrators		
	2.2 Understand the roles and boundaries of all workers with regard to the safe handling of medicines (prescribing, dispensing, administration, storage and disposal) in various contexts, for example: ■ Care homes (personal or nursing care) ■ Day services ■ An individual's own home ■ Sheltered accommodation ■ Supported housing ■ Other networks and services for individuals (education, religious establishments, voluntary agencies, activities and entertainment)		
	2.3 Understand the need to check that the medicine received matches the medication and dosage prescribed by the clinician and is listed on the appropriate documentation.		
	2.4 Understand the need to seek guidance and support (and from where) about the medicine and dosage prescribed for any particular individual, e.g. prescriber (medical or non-medical), NHS Direct, manager, nurse, or from supportive reference material.		
	2.5 Understand the need for confidentiality, when and to whom information about an individual's medication may be disclosed or discussed, e.g. doctor, pharmacist, other care professionals, relatives/solicitor with enduring power of attorney.		

Main area	Learning outcome	Learning outcome achieved (manager's or trainer's signature)	Date
3. Types of medicine and routes of administration	3.1 Understand the importance of some types of medication prescribed and administered to individuals, for example: ■ Antibiotics (used to fight infection) ■ Analgesics (used to relieve pain) ■ Anti-histamines (used to relieve allergy symptoms, e.g. hay fever) ■ Antacids (used to relieve indigestion) ■ Anti-coagulants (used to prevent blood clotting, e.g. following heart attack, thrombosis, some surgical procedures) ■ Psychotropic medicines (e.g. used to treat depression) ■ Diuretics (used to get rid of excess fluids in the body) ■ Laxatives (used to alleviate constipation) ■ Hormones (e.g. insulin, steroids, Hormone Replacement Therapy) ■ Cytotoxic medicines (used to treat some forms of cancer)		
	3.2 Understand the classification of medication: ■ Prescription only medicine (POM) ■ Over-the-counter medicine (P – in the presence of pharmacist; GSL – General Sales List) ■ Controlled Drugs ■ Complementary/homeopathic remedies		
	3.3 Understand the different routes by which medicines are administered and by whom: ■ Inhalation (use of inhalers – nasal or oral) ■ Injection (by piercing the skin) ■ Ingestion (medicines/tablets taken orally, including under the tongue)		

Main area	Learning outcome	Learning outcome achieved (manager's or trainer's signature)	Date
	- Topical (application of creams, lotions, ointments) - Infusion (intravenous drips) - Instillation (administration of drops to ears, nose/eyes) - PR – *per rectum* (enemas, suppositories) - PV – *per vagina* (pessaries, creams)		
	3.4 Understand the importance of noting and reporting any changes to an individual following administration of medicines. Some examples of symptoms of adverse reactions (long-term/short-term) may be: - Rashes - Breathing difficulties - Swellings - Nausea - Vomiting - Diarrhoea - Stiffness - Shaking - Headaches - Drowsiness - Constipation - Weight gain		
	3.5 Understand the need to check contraindications and medicine interactions prior to administration of home remedies or over-the-counter medicines, and complementary medicines and preparations.		

Main area	Learning outcome	Learning outcome achieved (manager's or trainer's signature)	Date
4. Safe practice in the administration of medicines	4.1 Understand the need to obtain the individual's consent* (and where applicable privacy) prior to administering medicines to them (includes invasive techniques such as administering suppositories). 1. *Where possible the individual provides informed consent. 2. When required the individual is provided with assistance to enable informed consent to take place (independent advocate, family member, medical professional) 3. If it is impossible to obtain informed consent, as many key people (independent advocates, family members and medical professionals) as possible act in the best interest of the individual.		
	4.2 Understand the need to carry out a risk assessment for each individual requiring medication in relation to: ■ Self-administration ■ Secondary administration of medicines by carer/family/friend or care worker		
	4.3 Understand the need for appropriate preparation prior to administering medicines: ■ Basic hygiene procedures ■ Having the correct equipment (e.g. gloves) ■ Having the correct recording documents available		
	4.4 Understand the need to ensure that the correct dose, of the correct medication, is given to the correct person at the correct time by the correct route or method.		

Main area	Learning outcome	Learning outcome achieved (manager's or trainer's signature)	Date
	4.5 Understand the need to correctly record: ■ The medication given ■ To whom the medication is given ■ The time it is given ■ The dosage given ■ The method of administration ■ Comments and signature after each administration		
	4.6 Understand the need to report and seek advice: ■ About reactions ■ About an individual's refusal to take medication ■ When errors in administration of the medicine occur (e.g. incorrect dose, incorrect medicine, to wrong individual, etc.)		
	4.7 Understand the requirements for careful and planned audits of medicine stock and its storage in accordance with the manufacturer's instructions and organisational policies: ■ Clean, ordered and secure environment ■ Correct temperature ■ Number of doses received, administered and remaining ■ Checking records for accuracy		
	4.8 Understand the need for the prompt and safe disposal of unwanted or out-of-date medicines.		

THE LIBRARY
TOWER HAMLETS COLLEGE
POPLAR HIGH STREET
LONDON E14 0AF
Tel: 0207 510 7763

Appendix 1 Blank MAR chart

MEDICATION ADMINISTRATION RECORD SHEETS

NAME				D.O.B.	
ALLERGIES				DOCTOR	
ADDRESS					
START DATE		PERIOD		START DAY	

			COMMENCING	WEEK 1								WEEK 2							WEEK 3							WEEK 4						
	MEDICATION DETAILS		DATE	28	27	26	25	24	23	22	21	20	19	18	17	16	15	14	13	12	11	10	9	8	7	6	5	4	3	2	1
			HOUR : DOSE																													
			M																													
			N																													
			T																													
			B																													
received	quant.	by	returned				quant.			by			destroyed				quant.			by											

(The above medication block repeats six times down the sheet, each with rows M, N, T, B and a received / quant. / by / returned / quant. / by / destroyed / quant. / by footer row.)

A - refused   B - nausea or vomiting   C - hospitalised   D - social leave   E - refused & destroyed

F - other (define)

A MAR chart

Appendix 2 Blank prescription

Pharmacy stamp	Age	Title, Forename, Surname & Address
	D.o.B	
Try not to stamp over age box		

Number of days' treatment N.B. Ensure dose is stated		NHS Number:

Endorsements

Signature of Prescriber   Date

For dispenser No. of Prescns. on form

NHS   PATIENTS – please read the notes overleaf

Appendix 3 Staff drug audit template

How to use this audit sheet

Managers should assess their staff to confirm they are competent in medicine administration and recording.

1. An audit must be completed on five drugs (one in MDS and, if possible, a Controlled Drug) prior to the drug round. The audit should be carried out without the care worker knowing it is taking place. This will establish a baseline that can be used to assess the care worker against.

2. It does not matter if this is not the calculated quantity the care setting should have, but it will highlight if there are any problems.

3. The manager should then repeat the drug audit directly after the drug round.

4. Appropriate action MUST be taken if discrepancies are found.

5. The returns book (in relation to the MAR chart) should be checked on a monthly basis to see if quantities tally.

A blank staff drug audit template can be found on page 101. The audit shown on page 102 demonstrates how the template should be used.

Staff drug audit

Name of staff member _____

DATE	TIME	NAME OF SERVICE USER	MEDICINE	DOSE	QUANTITY RECEIVED	QUANTITY RECORDED AS ADMINISTERED	CALCULATED QUANTITY	ACTUAL QUANTITY	✓ OR x
	before								
	after								
	before								
	after								
	before								
	after								
	before								
	after								
	before								
	after								

Staff drug audit (completed example)

Name of staff member ___ *A care assistant*

DATE	TIME	NAME OF SERVICE USER	MEDICINE	DOSE	QUANTITY RECEIVED	QUANTITY RECORDED AS ADMINISTERED	CALCULATED QUANTITY	ACTUAL QUANTITY	√ OR x
20.10.06	10am before	Joe Bloggs	Aspirin	75 mg 1 m	28	12	16	16	√
	10.30am after				28	12 + 1	16 - 1 = 15	15	√
20.10.06	10am before	Joe Bloggs	Sodium Valproate	200 mg 2 tds	84	44	40	42	x
	10.30am after				84	44 + 2	42 – 2 = 40	40	√
20.10.06	10am before	Edna Green	Amoxicillin	250 mg 1 tds	21	14	7	7	√
	10.30am after				21	14 + 1	7 - 1 = 6	7	x
20.10.06	10am before	Ivy Brown	Diazepam	5 mg 1 m	50	28	22	12	x
	10.30am after				50	28 + 1	12 – 1 =11	9	x
20.10.06	10am before	John Smith	Paracetamol	500 mg 1-2 prn	100	45	55	60	x
	10.30am after				100	45 + 1	60 - 1 =59	59	√

Glossary

Administer   to give or apply medicines to an individual

Audit trail   a record that can trace the exact usage of medicines

BNF   British National Formulary; a reference source that provides up to date guidance on the prescribing, dispensing and administration of medicines

Capacity   the ability to make informed decisions

Clinician   a doctor or nurse who can make decisions about the health of an individual

Compliance   the accuracy with which an individual takes their medication as prescribed

Concordance   the shared agreement between an individual and health care workers regarding the medication the individual has been prescribed, i.e. the individual knowing what medication they have been prescribed, what it is for and whether or not they want to take it

Confidentiality   keeping information secret and only discussing it with other people who have a right to know

Consent   the permission/agreement of an individual to receive medication administered to them

Contraindication   a sign, symptom or medical condition that indicates that a certain drug or other intervention should not be used

Controlled Drug   medicines that can be misused, such as those containing morphine. There are tight controls over the prescribing, dispensing and administration of Controlled Drugs

Covertly   secretively

Dispense   the supply of medicine to an individual by a pharmacist or dispensing doctor

Formulation   the way a medicine is made, which determines the route of administration, e.g. oral formulation

GSL   General Sales List medicine; a medicine that does not have to be prescribed by a medically trained person or dispensed by a pharmacist. A GSL medicine can be brought in shops etc. and include medicines such as paracetamol

Guidance documents   information detailing best practice

Home remedies   medicines that can be purchased over the counter for minor ailments

Indication   a sign, symptom or medical condition that indicates that a certain drug or other intervention should be used

Individual   the service user, patient or person in your care

Legislation   acts and regulations that make up the law. Legislation relating to medicines is there to protect you and the individuals you look after

MAR chart   Medication Administration Record chart; an official document that details the administration of medicines to an individual

MDS   Monitored Dosage System; the supply of an individual's medicines from a pharmacist in blister packs that show the time and date they should be taken

MIMS   Monthly Index of Medical Specialities; a reference source that provides information on medicines that are available on prescription and sold over the counter

NMS   National Minimum Standards; the minimum standards a service is expected to achieve to ensure good practice. NMS are supported by regulations

P   Pharmacy only medicines; medicines that can only be sold by a registered pharmacist

PIL   Product Information Leaflet; a leaflet that is provided by the pharmacist for each medicine dispensed. The PIL is written by the manufacturer and gives information about the ingredients in the medicine, the dose, how to take the medicine, any side effects etc.

Policy   a written document that outlines what should be done in certain circumstances within an organisation/company

POM   Prescription Only Medicines; medicines that can only be obtained by prescription

Prescribe   instructions from a medically trained person to a pharmacist to dispense a medicine or other intervention (e.g. a piece of equipment such as a support stocking). The type, amount and use of the medicine/intervention will be included

Prescription tax   the charge made for a NHS prescription; as of 1 April 2006, the charge for one item is £6.65

Prosecute   to charge an individual, company or organisation with committing a crime and start legal proceedings against them

Protocol   set of rules and reasons detailing how something is done

Regulations   rules that have to be followed

Side effect   an unwanted reaction caused by the taking of a medicine (e.g. nausea, rash, headache)

Verbal order   a request to change a treatment that is not made in writing, for example over the telephone

Index

abbreviations on prescriptions 19
Access to Health Records Act (1990) 8
Acts of Parliament 2–9
Administration and Control of Medicines,
    guidance document 10–11
administration of medicines 24–5
    by infusion 47
    by ingestion 44–5
    by inhalation 45
    by injection 46
    by instillation 47
    by PEG tube 49
    errors in 66–7
    recording correctly 62–5
    rectally 48
    safety procedures 58–9
    self-administration 56–7
    topically 46–7
    transdermally 48
    vaginally 48
adverse reactions to medication 50–1
alternative medicines 42
audits 68–9, 100–2

British National Formulary (BNF) 34

Care Standards Act (2000) 6
CD (Controlled Drugs) Register 43, 64
Chinese medicines 43
classification of medicine 42–3
cleaning fluids, safe labelling of 5
clinical waste, disposing safely 4, 70–1
complementary medicines 42
compliance checks 56, 57, 60
concordance 60
confidentiality 8–9, 38–9
consent see informed consent
contra indications, checking 52–3
Controlled Drugs (CDs) 43, 64–5, 70
COSHH (Control of Substances Hazardous
    to Health Regulations) 4
crushing tablets, problems with 44–5, 49

Data Protection Act (1998) 8
decisions about medication 6

dispensing of medication 3, 24–5
disposal of medicines 4, 70–1
dosages of medication
    changing after verbal orders 32–3
    knowledge of 40–1
drops, administering 47
drug audits 100–2

errors in drug administration 66–7

generic versus trade names 42
GSL (General Sales List) medicines 42
guidance documents 10–11

handling medicines, staff responsible for
    16–17
handwashing 59
harmful substances, storage of 4–5
Hazardous Waste Regulations (2005) 4
Health and Safety at Work Act (1974) 4
herbal medicines 42–3
home remedies 52–3
homeopathic medicines 42
hygiene procedures 58–9

identification of individuals 60–1
information sources on medicines 34–7
informed consent 54–5
infusion of medicines 47
ingestion of medicines 44–5
inhalation of medicines 45
injection of medicines 46
instillation of medicines 47
insulin injections 46

jargon on prescriptions 19

labelling of medicines 5, 24
legislation
    care standards 6
    decision-making capacity 6
    patient records 8
    relating to medicines 2–3
    workplace safety 4–5

MAR charts 26–9, 32, 62–5, 98
MDS (Monitored Dosage Systems) 24–5
medical records, access to 8
medication
    dose changes 32–3
    legislation 2–3
    for new individuals 30–1
    policies/procedures 12–13
    self-administration 56–7
    ways of administering 44–9
Medicine Administration Record (MAR)
    charts *see* MAR charts
medicines
    audits of stock 68–9
    classification of 42–3
    dispensing of 24–5
    information sources 34–7
    knowledge of 40–1
    labelling of 24
    receipt of 24–5
    responsibility for handling 16–17
    safe disposal of 70–1
    side effects of 36–7, 40–1, 50–1
    storage of 68–9
    types of 40–3
Medicines Act (1968) 3, 20, 42, 44
Medicines (Labelling) Regulations (1976) 24
Mental Capacity Act (2005) 6, 55
MIMS (Monthly Index of Medical
    Specialities) 34
Misuse of Drugs Act (1971) 3, 43
Misuse of Drugs (Safe Custody) Regulations
    (1973) 3, 43
Monitored Dosage Systems (MDS) 24–5

National Minimum Standards (NMS) 6, 7, 12
new individuals' medications 30–1

ointments, applying 46
oral medication, administering 44–5
over-the-counter medicines 52–3

patient consent 54–5
patient records, confidentiality of 8–9

PEG (Percutaneous Endoscopic
    Gastrostomy) 49
PIL (Product Information Leaflet) 34
policies and procedures 12–13
POM (Prescription Only Medicines) 42
prescriptions
    blank prescription 99
    checking 18
    jargon used 19
    Medicines Act (1968) 3, 20
    ordering 21–3
    recording on MAR chart 26–9
    signing back of 20
Product Information Leaflet (PIL) 34

recording medication given 62–5
rectal medicines 48
register of controlled drugs 43, 64
regulations 2–11
reporting errors 66–7
risk assessments 56–7
roles and responsibilities of staff 14–17

seeking advice 66–7
self-administration of medication 56–7
side effects of medication 36–7, 40–1, 50–1
skin patches 48
sources of information 34–7
staff drug audits 68–9, 100–2
staff roles and responsibilities 14–17
storage of medicines 3, 68–9

topical application of medicines 46–7
trade *versus* generic names 42
transdermal medicines 48

unwanted medicines, disposal of 4, 70–1

vaginal medicines 48
verbal orders, recording dose changes
    32–3

waste disposal 4, 70–1
workplace safety laws 4